W0230674

Transcultural Care

Transcultural Care

A Book and Video Guide to Cultural Competence in Healthcare Professions

Irena Papadopoulos

PhD, MA (Ed), BA, DipNEd, DipN, NDN, RCM, RGN, RNT, FHEA, FETNA
Professor of Transcultural Health and Nursing
Head, Research Centre for Transcultural Studies in Health
School of Health and Education
Middlesex University
London, UK

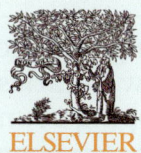

ELSEVIER

Copyright 2026, by Elsevier Limited. All rights are reserved, including those for text and data mining, AI training, and similar technologies.

For accessibility purposes, images in electronic versions of this book are accompanied by alt text descriptions provided by Elsevier. For more information, see https://www.elsevier.com/about/accessibility.

Publisher's note: *Elsevier* takes a neutral position with respect to territorial disputes or jurisdictional claims in its published content, including in maps and institutional affiliations.

The right of Irena Papadopoulos to be identified as author of this work has been asserted by her in accordance with the Copyright, Designs and Patents Act 1988.

No part of this publication may be reproduced or transmitted in any form or by any means, electronic or mechanical, including photocopying, recording, or any information storage and retrieval system, without permission in writing from the publisher. Details on how to seek permission, further information about the Publisher's permissions policies, and our arrangements with organizations such as the Copyright Clearance Center and the Copyright Licensing Agency can be found at our website: www.elsevier.com/permissions.

This book and the individual contributions contained in it are protected under copyright by the Publisher (other than as may be noted herein).

Notice
Practitioners and researchers must always rely on their own experience and knowledge in evaluating and using any information, methods, compounds, or experiments described herein. Because of rapid advances in the medical sciences, in particular, independent verification of diagnoses and drug dosages should be made. To the fullest extent of the law, no responsibility is assumed by Elsevier, authors, editors, or contributors for any injury and/or damage to persons or property as a matter of products liability, negligence, or otherwise, or from any use or operation of any methods, products, instructions, or ideas contained in the material herein.

ISBN: 978-0-443-12667-3

Content Strategist: Trinity Hutton & Jennifer Dooley
Content Project Manager: Piyush Mohan Bhatnagar
Design: Greg Harris
Marketing Manager: Deborah Watkins

Printed in India
Last digit is the print number: 9 8 7 6 5 4 3 2 1

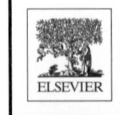

Working together to grow libraries in developing countries

www.elsevier.com • www.bookaid.org

Contents

List of Online Videos

Videos are available at Evolve, visit evolve.elsevier.com

About the Author

Dr Irena Papadopoulos is the former Head of the Research Centre for Transcultural Studies in Health (established in 1995), former Chair of her School's Ethics Committee, former Chair of the research team for Nursing, Midwifery and Allied Health Professions, and co-founder of ETNA (European Transcultural Nurses Association). She is the leading partner of the research which led to the development of Papadopoulos, Tilki and Taylor (PTT) model for cultural competence (1998), which she has expanded in 2006 and 2018. This pioneering model has been widely adopted worldwide along with her assessment tool for measuring cultural competence (CCA-Tool). In 2007, she co-founded the *Intercultural Education for Nurses in Europe* (IENE) program, which includes 11 EU-funded projects. In 2015, she established the *International Culturally Competent and Compassionate Online Surveys* (ICC-COS) program, bringing together researchers from 25 countries to conduct global studies on cultural competence and compassion in healthcare. During 2017-2021 she led the CARESSES's project (HORIZON) development of the conceptual framework, guidelines and content for the creating and programming of the first culturally competent socially assistive robot. Over the years she recevied a number of awards such as Finalist for the *Madame Figaro* (Cyprus) woman scientist of the year (2013 & 2017), the Middlesex University staff 'Best Research Impact' (2016), and 'Project of the Year' in 2018 and 2019, winner of the outstanding article of the year by Emerald Publishing Company (2018), winner of the 2023 international book PROSE award, winner of the *Journal of Research in Nursing* (JRN) Veronica Bishop article of the year (2023). She has authored a number of books and hunderds of articles, keynotes, master classes, and open access materials.

Foreword

When reflecting on the historical development of transcultural nursing, one cannot overlook how global societal changes have shaped the path of nursing education. What once began as a marginal or even overlooked component is now a central pillar in preparing nurses to provide safe, respectful, and equitable care in multicultural societies.

This change has not happened on its own. It is the result of a growing awareness that healthcare professionals must take into account the cultural background, beliefs, and lived realities of each individual patient if it is to be truly person-centered. In recent decades, increasing global migration, geopolitical instability, and growing health inequalities have emphasized the urgency of equipping healthcare professionals with cultural competence. The resulting cultural complexity of healthcare has made it abundantly clear that culturally competent care is not a privilege, but a human right.

Nursing education systems have had to respond to this, and they have. Curricula are increasingly incorporating transcultural principles, both through formal courses and through practical learning. However, this progress is due to pioneers who foresaw this change long before it was widely accepted. Professor Irena Papadopoulos stands out among them. Her scholarly contributions, practical framework, and persistent advocacy have laid the intellectual and ethical foundation for a model of care that honors human diversity in all its dimensions.

This book continues this legacy. It offers a timely and necessary examination of transcultural nursing, not as a static concept, but as a living evolving practice—a practice shaped not only by education, context, and engagement but also by the ongoing transformation of societies, emerging technologies, and the changing realities of global health systems. It not only builds on decades of theoretical and practical work in transcultural nursing but also expands the discussion into new and urgent areas that need to be addressed. By incorporating concepts such as virtuous leadership, technological innovation, and even the ethical relationship between human and nonhuman beings, it challenges readers to reconceptualize cultural competence for the realities of the 21st century and beyond.

Organized into six interconnected chapters, the book takes the reader from a foundational understanding of culture and its importance in healthcare, through theoretical frameworks and conceptual pillars, to advanced and timely topics such as culturally competent leadership, culturally competent and compassionate spiritual care, and the impact of artificial intelligence and robotics on culturally competent practice. Each chapter is clearly written and intellectually rich, offering practical examples, clear definitions, and reflective insights that engage the reader not only cognitively but also personally and ethically. Due to its structure and clarity, this book is suitable not only for undergraduate and postgraduate education but also for use in continuing education programs and clinical training. It is also relevant for policymakers, healthcare managers, and anyone involved in the design of culturally appropriate services.

What makes this book particularly valuable is its balance between philosophical depth and pedagogical clarity. The "Big Six Cs"—communication, compassion, courage, collaboration, cybernetics, and connectivity—form a unique and memorable framework that combines timeless values with modern challenges. Equally noteworthy is the author's bold inclusion of posthumanist thought and nonhuman actors, extending the conventional boundaries of cultural competence into ethically and technologically complex terrain.

The integration of personal narratives, cultural history, and applicable models results in a multidimensional and transformative learning experience. The reader is challenged not only to understand cultural competence but also to reflect on it, internalize it, and live it as a dynamic and lifelong moral commitment. Therefore, this is not a conventional book, but a compelling interdisciplinary resource that bridges theory and practice, past and future, insight and action. Professor Papadopoulos, with her meticulous attention to detail and far-reaching vision for the future of transcultural nursing, has created a work that is scholarly yet accessible, visionary yet grounded. Her ability to make complex ideas both understandable and usable, supported by visualizations and real-life cases, makes this book an indispensable resource for students, teachers, researchers, and healthcare professionals working toward equitable and compassionate care.

Mirko Prosen
PhD, MSc, BSc, RN, FFNMRCSI
Senior Research Associate, Associate Professor,
Vice-dean for Students Affairs, President of the
University of Primorska Alumni Club

Foreword

Healthcare around the world is more complex than ever, not only in terms of diseases and their treatments but also in terms of patients from different ethnic and cultural backgrounds, advances in technology, and so on. No matter how complex and overwhelming things have become in healthcare, our mission is to provide quality care to all people, regardless of where you work, who the patients are, and where they come from. Everyone has the right to access affordable, quality, and appropriate healthcare and to be treated with respect and dignity. To achieve this, we, as healthcare professionals, must be able to care for our clients with respect, relieve their pain, comfort them, and reassure them of their quality of life from birth to death. What skills do we need to provide culturally appropriate care, and how can we acquire them? Cultural competence in the health profession does not always come naturally; it must be learned and developed throughout one's professional career. This book will pave the way for you to provide culturally appropriate care to all the clients who come to you from all over the world.

The author of this book is Professor Irena Papadopoulos, president of the European Transcultural Nursing Association. She has been leading and inspiring healthcare researchers and practitioners worldwide for many years. She developed "The Papadopoulos Model of Cultural Competence," which is presented in this book and also in her other work, "Transcultural Health and Social Care—Development of Culturally Competent Practitioners," published in 2006. In her earlier book, she described how "transcultural or cultural competence constitutes a health and social care imperative in the 21st century." What is remarkable about her theory is that she has a bird's-eye view of cultures and religions, from the United Kingdom and Europe to the Far East, where I am from, as well as the world at large, along with a deep knowledge and compassion for them. From this book, you will learn the knowledge and skills that lead to transcultural competence, as well as an attitude of compassion.

Transcultural nursing has been known to nurses since Dr. Madeleine Leininger began her efforts to develop the "Sunrise Model" in the mid-1950s. Since then, our circumstances have changed drastically so that now, when we talk about "transcultural nursing," we must consider not only people's culture and ethnicity but also all types of people, including immigrants, refugees, and asylum seekers. We must further take into account noncommunicable diseases, emerging, reemerging, and neglected infectious diseases, climate change, planetary health, and the health inequalities caused by all of these.

This book will guide you through the world of transcultural nursing through history, including what we have learned from ancient wisdom to the present world through the COVID-19 pandemic. You will not only acquire knowledge about cultural competence but can go further and become a culturally competent leader as well. This book's uniqueness lies in its description of culturally competent and virtuous leadership; you will not be able to learn it anywhere else. For example, the chapter "Culturally Competent and Compassionate Spiritual Care: Lessons From the COVID-19 Pandemic" presents how important and helpful spiritual care was to us during this difficult time, including descriptions from Professor Papadopoulos's dedicated research. After reading this book, I am sure you will be more confident and skilled in providing culturally congruent care and will strive to be a leader in improving nursing care for all people.

I hope that you enjoy this book and that you continue to expand the frontier for nursing care worldwide. Please enjoy your journey into transcultural nursing.

It is a great honor for me to write the foreword for this wonderful book by Irena.

Tomiko Toda
Associate Professor
Otemae University
Osaka, Japan
April 2025

Foreword

The discovery of social determinants of health has unraveled the impact of social, political, and environmental conditions on the well-being of populations across the globe. Culturally diverse groups have greater exposure to adverse social determinants through systemic discrimination, exclusion, and marginalization resulting in cumulative social disadvantages reflected in poorer physical and mental health. Cultural competence in healthcare, policymaking, and leadership is imperative to promote health equity.

Professor Papadopoulos, a renowned international scholar, educator, researcher, leader, and author in Transcultural Nursing and Social Care, has written this book to underscore the role of cultural competence in promoting health equity. Her model explicates cultural competence as a process of development grounded in the social structural realities that reproduce social and health inequities in society. This model emphasizes compassion as the emotional and cognitive connection with the plight of the socially disadvantaged that can move others toward culturally competent actions to achieve health equity.

Professor Papadopoulos is a pioneer in collaborative design of socially assistive robots imbued with humanistic characteristics for elder care. This book represents an innovative expansion of cultural competence built upon connectivity between humans and technology. It is for certain that technological advances will continue and collaborative expertise between health and technology professionals will be required to expand its application in healthcare. Increased population diversity worldwide will necessitate use of assistive technologies that are culturally competent.

The author introduces the "Big Six Cs" of *communication*, *compassion*, *courage*, *collaboration*, *cybernetics*, and *connectivity* as the futuristic and pragmatic pathway for integrating technology to enhance culturally competent and humanistic care for diverse populations. In fact, there are plenty of examples of technological applications in healthcare, such as artificial intelligence–enhanced diagnosis, data-driven decision-making, digital health, and wearable technology, and in genomics. Population diversity will require technological assistance with communication using different languages. The COVID-19 pandemic heightened the need for connectivity by isolated patients and with their significant others. Bold, creative, and courageous leadership can forge collaboration with other experts to design technology to enhance human care.

The book offers a visionary posthumanism perspective premised on the coexistence of humans and technology as inherent to our future. It challenges the status quo of exclusion and fear of technology as essentially inhumane. It argues for a new understanding and acceptance of technology as integral to life. It challenges multidisciplinary students, professionals, administrators, and educators to examine technological advancements as endemic to humanity and adapt technology to improve health of individuals and populations. The author's work with socially assistive robotics gives credence to her ability to adapt technology to enhance transcultural and culturally competent healthcare.

Dula F. Pacquiao, EdD, RN, CTN-A, FTNSS, FNYAM
Professor Emerita
Rutgers, the State University of New Jersey, USA

Preface

It is with great pleasure that I present to you my new book, 'Transcultural Care: A Book and Video Guide to Cultural Competence in Healthcare Professions'. This book is the culmination of my 40-year journey of learning, researching, teaching, and practicing cultural competence in the field of nursing.

Nineteen years have passed since the publication of my last English book on transcultural nursing and cultural competence in 2006, which expanded and modified the original 1998 book which introduced the Papadopoulos, Tilki, and Taylor model of transcultural nursing. The 2006 book provided the pillars and principles of the model and offered an international perspective on the field of transcultural nursing.

Now, in the 21st century, the importance of cultural competence has become more evident than ever. This new book focuses on the significance of cultural competence in today's world, introducing new elements such as compassion and theories such as that of posthumanism. It emphasizes the connection of cultural competence for humans with that of nonhuman entities and the environment.

The book is divided into six chapters, each exploring different aspects of cultural competence. Chapter 1 discusses culture and its relevance to health and care, while Chapter 2 delves into cultural competence for the 21st century. Chapter 3 introduces the key concepts, which I call the 'Big Six Cs': Communication, Compassion, Courage, Collaboration, Cybernetics, and Connectivity. Chapter 4 explores culturally competent and virtuous leadership, and Chapter 5 provides lessons from the COVID-19 pandemic on culturally competent and compassionate spiritual care. Finally, Chapter 6 examines the implications of cultural competence in AI and robotics for healthcare and nursing.

A unique feature of this book is the inclusion of information from ancient to modern eras in every chapter, adopting philosophical and technological perspectives from different cultures. This approach reflects my belief in the importance of understanding the historical and cultural contexts that shaped our understanding of cultural competence in our era and hopefully will guide the future generations. Albert Einstein is credited as the person who spoke these wise words: 'Learn from yesterday, live for today, hope for tomorrow. The important thing is not to stop questioning.' The American astronomer, planetary scientist, and science communicator Carl Sagan (1934–1996) declared, 'You have to know the past to understand the present.'

Writing this book has been a deeply personal and rewarding experience, allowing me to reflect on the many lessons I have learned throughout my career. It is my sincere hope that this book will contribute to the ongoing conversation about cultural competence in nursing and healthcare and inspire readers to embrace cultural competence as an essential component of their practice.

As you read this book, I invite you to reflect on your own experiences and consider how you can apply the principles of cultural competence in your own practice. Together, we can work towards creating a more inclusive, compassionate, and culturally competent healthcare system that meets the needs of all individuals and communities.

Irena Papadopoulos

Dedication

To my beloved husband.
For walking beside me for more than five
decades, and for encouraging and believing in
me. Your unwavering support has made this
book, and many others, possible.

Chapter 1

Culture and Its Relevance in Health and Care

Learning Objectives

After reading this chapter you should:

- Become aware of influence of culture on health.
- Appreciate the various influences on culture and cultural change.
- Learn about some cultural theories.
- Gain a historical perspective and definitions of culture.
- Expand your knowledge about cultural identity.
- Reflect on the impact of culture on health and well-being.

Introduction

I owe my love of celestial space, culture, and technology to the TV series *Star Trek*.

In the 23rd century, Captain Kirk often encountered alien cultures and civilizations during his missions. He believed that understanding and respecting other cultures were essential to building peaceful relationships and cooperation between 'species'.

We are not living in the 23rd century. In our 21st century, it is unlikely that we will encounter alien cultures; nevertheless, the statement of Captain Kirk is very relevant to us today. All we need to do is to replace the word "species" with "cultures."

In this chapter, I aim to outline some key notions related to culture and cultural identity. We are all members of a culture and most likely, in our era, may belong to more than one culture. I also aim to explore the impact that culture and cultural identity have on our health and the way the care establishments provide their services.

We will remind ourselves that culture is a dynamic global concept that is influenced by a number of powerful factors and the rapidly changing world.

It is, however, impossible to provide the colossal corpus of knowledge in one chapter. A plethora of books and articles have been written about culture from numerous perspectives, many of which are on open access on the Internet, so if you wish to learn more than what this chapter can offer, it will not be too hard.

Everyone Is Talking About Culture

Culture is a complex and multifaceted concept that has been defined in various ways by different scholars and thinkers throughout the centuries. These days the notion of culture is very popular, and it is sprinkled generously during conversations with family members, friends, work colleagues, customers, providers of services, and so on. If asked, each one of us will define culture in their own way depending on their age, gender, religion, worldviews, education, life experiences, personal priorities, where in the world they live, and more.

In my 2006 book on transcultural health and social care, I defined culture in the following way:

All human beings are cultural beings. Culture is the shared way of life of a group of people that includes beliefs, values, ideas, language, communication, norms, and visibly expressed forms, such as customs, art, music, clothing and etiquette. Culture influences individuals' lifestyles, personal identity and their relationship with others, both within and outside their culture. Cultures are dynamic and ever changing as individuals are influenced by it as well as influence it, in different degrees.

Papadopoulos, 2006, p. 10

It is because of the dynamic nature of culture that today I would define culture slightly differently.

The popularity of culture as a topic of discussion in recent years is due to a number of reasons such as:

Identity and belonging: As people increasingly seek to define their own identities and find a sense of belonging in a rapidly changing world, culture has become an important part of that process. People are looking to connect with others who share their cultural heritage or values and are exploring different cultural traditions and practices.

Workplace diversity: Companies are recognizing the benefits of having a diverse workforce and are actively seeking to recruit employees from different backgrounds. This has led to a greater focus on understanding and managing different cultures in the workplace.

Global economics: Big companies, especially the global giants, are realizing that understanding their customers' cultures helps them modify their products and their marketing strategies to the sensitivities of each culture, thus enabling them to be more acceptable and, of course, more profitable.

Globalization: With the increasing interconnectedness of the world through technology, trade, social media, and travel, people are encountering other cultures more frequently than ever before. This has led to a greater awareness and appreciation of cultural diversity.

Sociopolitical issues: A number of social and political issues in recent years have brought culture and cultural differences to the forefront of public discourse. Examples include the Black Lives Matter movement, the #MeToo movement, and debates over immigration and multiculturalism.

The summary of key points is provided in the box below.

Summary of Key Points

- Culture is a complex and multifaceted concept that has been defined in various ways by different scholars and thinkers throughout the centuries.
- The popularity of culture as a topic of discussion in recent years is due to:
  - Identity and belonging
  - Workplace diversity

- Global economics
- Globalization
- Sociopolitical issues

Walking Through the Centuries of 'Culture' Definitions

Starting with the Greek philosopher Aristotle (384–322 BC), who explored the role of culture in shaping individual and social identity in his "Poetics" (Kenny, translator, 2013), we encounter his view of culture as the cultivation of human excellence and the pursuit of the good life. He believed that culture was a means of developing virtues such as wisdom, courage, compassion, and justice, all of which were essential for individual and societal well-being. Even before Aristotle, China's most famous teacher, philosopher, and political theorist, Confucius (551–479 BC), promoted the use of rituals that encouraged the benefits of respectful attitude and the creation of a sense of community within a group. A key teaching of Confucius was the notion of "filial piety," or devotion to family, which remains to this day a key cultural characteristic of the Chinese culture (Legge, translator, 1971).

During the first half of the first millennium, the Western world often understood culture in terms of the classical Greco-Roman tradition, which viewed culture as a range of intellectual and artistic pursuits, including philosophy, literature, music, and visual arts. Culture was seen as a means of achieving a higher level of civilization. Of importance in this era is the beginning of the dominance of Christianity. Religious beliefs and practices were often integrated into artistic and intellectual pursuits. For example, Saint Augustine (AD 354–430), a Christian theologian, emphasized the role of culture and education in shaping Christian beliefs and practices, declaring that culture is the means by which we understand and interpret the world around us, and it is through culture that we come to know God.

In other parts of the world, such as in East Asia, culture was often understood in a more holistic sense. In China and India—both huge and diverse countries—regional cultural practices existed, but in order to nurture their national cultural identities, countrywide festivals emerged, which brought people together. In China, in addition to the Chinese New Year/Spring Festival established in the previous era (c.1600–1046 BC), the Mid-Autumn Festival/Moon Festival started between AD 618 and 907. In India, in addition to the Diwali/Festival of Lights, which is believed to have originated during the years 1500–500 BC, the Holi/Festival of Colors became an India-wide event starting around AD 320–550.

Almost the whole of East Asia was developing cultures encompassing a wide range of activities and practices, including forms of martial arts, the use of traditional medicine, literature, music, philosophy, religion, art, and social customs. This understanding of culture emphasized the interconnectedness of different aspects of human experience, aimed at cultivating well-rounded and virtuous individuals.

In the Arabic-speaking countries, the teachings of Prophet Muhammad (AD 570–632), the founder of Islam, had a major impact, as culture was defined by the teachings of the Quran and the Hadith. These two holy books prescribed the traditions and practices of the early Islamic community. In addition, Islamic culture encompassed a wide range of intellectual and artistic pursuits, including philosophy, science, poetry, and architecture.

In other parts of the world, the Persian philosopher and physician Avicenna (AD 980–1037) wrote about culture and its impact on human behavior and society. He viewed culture as the force that shapes the way we think, feel, and act, adding that it is through culture that we are able to understand and appreciate the complexity of the world.

In the early 20th century in Europe and North America, culture was often associated with modernism and new and experimental ideas and methods in art, music, and literature, which rejected traditional forms of artistic expression in favor of experimentation and innovation. Culture was seen as a means of questioning and critiquing social norms and conventions. Anthropologists were making a major contribution with their research on culture. For example, the American anthropologist Margaret Mead (1901–1978) defined culture as a vital and indispensable element of a healthy society, while the British anthropologist Mary Douglas (1921–2007), known for her work on human culture and symbolism, declared that culture is a set of shared meanings and symbols that shape how we interpret and interact with the world around us.

Starting at the beginning of the 20th century, Australia and the United States welcomed thousands of European migrants who naturally took with them their cultural traditions, values, and beliefs. Both countries quickly became an amalgam of multiple cultures.

In other parts of the world, such as in Africa and Asia, culture was often associated with resistance to colonialism and imperialism, with a focus on reclaiming and preserving traditional cultural practices and identities. Culture was seen as a means of asserting political and cultural autonomy in the face of colonial domination.

Mahatma Gandhi (1869–1948), known for his philosophy of truth and nonviolence, led the movement for India's independence and defined culture as the widening of the mind and spirit to embrace all aspects of human life, including religion, art, literature, science, and politics. For Gandhi, culture was a source of inspiration and a means to achieve social and political transformation (Gandhi, 1932).

Nelson Mandela (1918–2013), the former South African president and anti-apartheid activist, viewed culture as a powerful tool for promoting social cohesion and nation-building. He saw culture as the mean of expressing the unique identity and values of a people and as a source of strength and resilience in the face of adversity (Mandela, 1995).

In the second half of the 20th century in Europe and the United States, culture is associated with consumerism and leisure activities involving, for example, radio, television, and cinema. As globalization became more prominent, more instances came to the fore of the early global and hybrid cultures that are about the mixing and blending of different cultural elements, such as customs, traditions, and beliefs, to create something new and unique. The impact of global cultures and cultural hybridization in the 20th century was significant. An example of global culture is the phenomenon of McDonalization (Ritzer, 1993), since most countries across the globe offer McDonald's fast food products, all of which are prepared and provided to the customers in the same way, although limited culture-specific products are also available in different countries.

In the posthuman 21st century, we find that definitions of culture, although similar with the previous human-oriented definitions, emphasize the importance of understanding culture in a broader context that includes nonhuman entities such as animals, machines, and the environment.

Having explored the various definitions of culture, I am now able to provide an adapted version of my original definition:

All human beings are cultural beings. Culture is the shared way of life of a group of people that includes beliefs, values, ideas, language, communication, norms, and visibly expressed forms, such as customs, art, music, clothing, and etiquette. Culture in a broader context includes nonhuman entities such as animals, machines, and the environment.

A frequent companion of "culture" are the notions of "race" and "ethnicity", the definition of which differ from that of "culture". According to Fernando (1991), "race" is a biological term and refers to physical appearance and genetic ancestry. The notion of race is controversial, as it has been used to create a taxonomy of human beings in order to abuse and exploit certain cultural groups. The terms "racism" and "racial prejudice" are closely linked to "race". Racism is an ideology about assumptions and value judgments about inferior and superior races of people, while dogma is about power and domination of the assumed inferior people.

Racial prejudice is a feeling or attitude of mind expressed as an antipathy based on faulty and inflexible generalizations and stereotypes. "Ethnicity" is generally defined as a sense of belonging, having similar physical appearance and social similarities.

The summary of key points is provided in the following box.

Summary of Key Points

- Understanding and respecting different cultures are key to building a more inclusive and harmonious world.
- Throughout the centuries, the notion of culture was described in both similar and different ways.
- Appreciating the history of culture enables us to understand the current cultures in broader and deeper ways.
- In the posthuman 21st century, we find that definitions of culture emphasize the importance of understanding culture in a broader context that includes nonhuman entities such as animals, machines, and the environment.

Outlining the Various Influences on Culture and Cultural Change

As you can see in Figure 1.1, a number of factors influence the development and ongoing changes of cultures. The geography of the place people live in has and continues to have a huge influence on the human culture. Some people live in mountainous areas, others live near the sea, and still others in desert-like lands. Each location has different climate, fauna and flora, and other aspects that impact all aspects of people's lives. For example, our

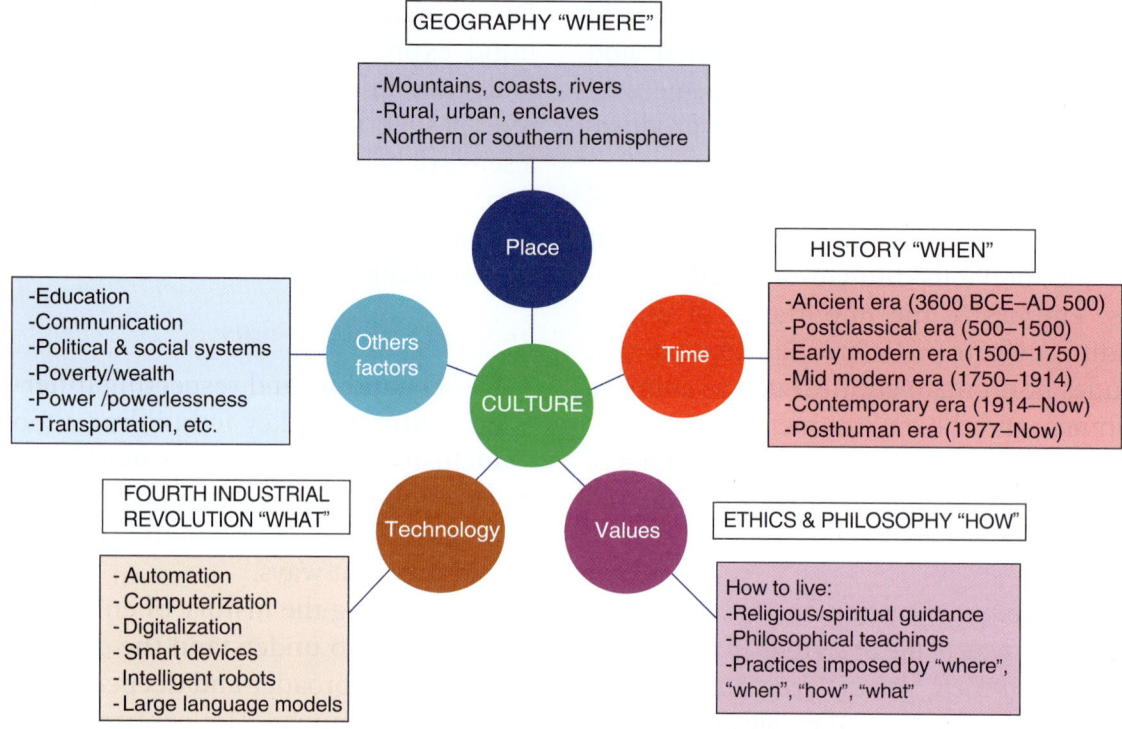

Figure 1.1 Influences on culture and cultural change.

ancestors sourced food sustainable in the geographical location they lived and subsequently developed ways of cooking, eating, and establishing customs and rituals around food. Although culture is continuously evolving, variations of these customs and practices are carried through generations.

Historical events over the centuries, such as wars, colonization, and so on, influenced the development of specific cultural attitudes toward patriotism, power, and peace (Woodward, 2007).

Ethics, philosophy, and religion contribute to the development of our values and the establishment of moral quotes and rituals in all cultures (Casanova, 2011).

More recently, the technological revolution has changed radically the work, social, commercial, and leisure cultures and much more. For example, we are currently experiencing major changes in communication practices. The rise of the Internet and smartphones has revolutionized the way people communicate. The proliferation of social media has given rise to a new culture of online interaction, where people can share information and ideas with anyone, anywhere in the world. The automation of many jobs through intelligent robots and computerization has changed the culture of the work environment, the nature of work, and the kinds of skills that are valued and has enabled people to work more flexibly and independently.

Other culture-influencing factors are the levels and types of education, politics and societal structures, as well as the existing large chasm between those living in poverty and those living with unbelievable levels of wealth.

The summary of key points is provided in the following box.

Summary of Key Points

- Factors influencing the development and ongoing changes of cultures are:
  - Place (Geography)
  - Time (History)
  - Values (Ethics and Philosophy)
  - Technology (Fourth Industrial Revolution, AI, and Robotics)
  - Other: Education, Political and Social Systems, Poverty/Wealth, Power/Powerlessness, Communication, Transportation, Health

Theories About Culture

THE CULTURAL ICEBERG THEORY

The American anthropologist Edward T. Hall built his popular theory of culture using the metaphor of an iceberg (Hall, 1984). According to his theory, there are three levels of culture. Level 1 is the tip of the iceberg, which represents the 5–10% of the visible level (also called the conscious level) of one's culture. This level provides cultural elements such as dress, language, food, rituals, and other cultural behaviors a person is conscious of and an observer can see. Beneath the visible part of the iceberg (the second level) lay the invisible or subconscious elements of culture, such as values, feelings, attitudes, beliefs, and principles, that we acquire through socialization from early childhood and adolescence, with further evolution during adulthood's life experiences. These are not visible to outsiders of the particular culture. Even individuals may not be aware of their own cultural elements that exist below the tip of the iceberg unless they reflect on their behaviors. My research on socially assistive robots adapted Hall's theory by adding the notion of "the trigger." It was important to develop a way through which the robot could observe and understand the hidden cultural elements in order to respond appropriately to those in its care. The observation study noted that unexpected events, such as receiving bad news (Figure 1.2), function as

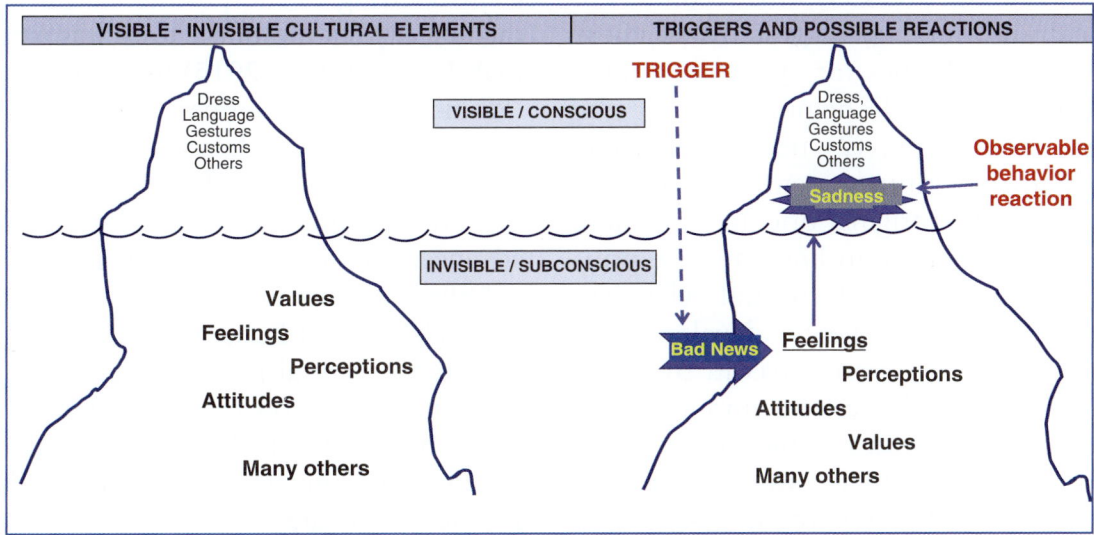

Figure 1.2 Cultural iceberg: Triggers and reactions.

triggers that stimulate element(s) situated in the invisible/subconscious part of the iceberg to move to the visible/conscious tip of the iceberg, thus creating observable behaviors, such as the expression(s) of sadness. We captured many triggers from people of different cultures and documented their responses. We found that there were cultural differences in the enactment of behaviors of the same or similar trigger (Papadopoulos & Koulouglioti, 2022).

The third level of culture lies at the deepest part of the iceberg. These are the implicit rules of the culture, known by all members of a cultural group but seldom stated.

THE THEORY OF CULTURAL RELATIVISM

All humans share fundamental values such as love, freedom, justice, growth, life, health, and security. However, these universal values are experienced and may be understood differently in different cultures. Health and social care is acceptable to members of specific groups if it respects their cultural values and is appropriate to their cultural needs. Leininger (1995), the founder of transcultural nursing, suggested that there are three possibilities for culturally appropriate healthcare: (1) helping preserve the cultural orientation; (2) negotiating some change in the cultural orientation; and (3) repatterning the original orientation. These three approaches are in line with the principles of the theory of cultural relativism (Boas, 1962). This theory, developed by the anthropologist Franz Boas in the early 20th century, emphasizes the importance of understanding cultures in their own terms, without judging them according to external standards. Cultural relativism asserts that every culture has its own unique values,

beliefs, and practices that are shaped by its history and social context.

Kavanagh and Kennedy (1992) stated that cultural relativism has its limitations. I frequently hear nursing students and other healthcare practitioners say that sometimes they disagree with the cultural beliefs and practices of their patients/clients but fear to challenge them to avoid being branded as racists. In my view, although cultural relativism is an appropriate theory to be used in the education of health and social care personnel, it must be balanced and supplemented by ethical debates and the development of culturally competent communication. It is crucial to understand the background and justification of dangerous cultural practices and be competent and compassionate in the way we communicate disagreement.

THE POSTHUMANIST THEORY AND CULTURE

It would be amiss on my part if I do not, albeit very briefly, include one of the most recent theories that is bound to impact health and social care practitioners and their workplaces. I am referring to the posthumanism theory, the first explicit use of the term was made by Ihab Hassan (1925–2015) in his 1977 essay, "Prometheus as Performer: Towards a Posthumanist Culture." Hassan described a shift in the understanding of human nature and the human condition in light of technological advancements and cultural changes.

Other posthumanist theorists such as Haraway (1985) and Braidotti (2013) sought to remove the central position occupied by the humans, aiming to expand our understanding of the world by including nonhuman entities such as animals, plants, and machines. Posthumanists argue that traditional anthropocentric views of culture and society are too limited and that we need to recognize the agency and importance of nonhuman entities in shaping human culture and society. This perspective emphasizes the interconnectedness of all living and nonliving entities and the need for a more ecological and holistic approach to understanding culture.

Posthumanism proposes that human beings can transcend their biological limitations through technology, such as the use of prosthetic limbs, pacemakers, and the use of artificial intelligence (AI) and robotics to perform surgery or provide assistance and companionship to people. During the COVID-19 pandemic, nurses and chaplains used smart devices to facilitate the communication between patients and their loved ones. AI assistants were also used by the bedside for patients to request and be provided with prayers, music, and other information without the involvement of the busy nurses. Telemedicine is increasingly being used to provide remote care to patients, such as remote consultations and telemonitoring. According to Schwab (2016), the Fourth Industrial Revolution is already changing how we live, work, and communicate. It is reshaping all aspects of government, such as education, healthcare, and commerce. It can change our relationships, our opportunities, and our identities as it changes the physical and virtual worlds we inhabit and even, in some cases, our bodies. In the future, it can also change the things we value and the way we value them.

Apart from technological devices, the benefits of animal therapies and their supportive care to humans are increasingly being appreciated. Animals provide companionship to adults and young children, especially those with anxiety disorders; they are trained to raise the alarm in an emergency; they can assist people in wheelchairs by fetching things; they act as guides to people with visual impairments; and so on.

It is inevitable that advanced technology will continue to be developed and embedded in all health and social care institutions. The benefits are gradually being recognized, but there remain many challenges and unsolved issues such as the transparency and ethics surrounding the use of the data being collected by AI devices and robots, concerns regarding malfunctions, their vulnerability to hacking, the legal agency of artificially intelligent robots and devices, and so on. Finally, almost all of these technologies are not culturally competent, apart from the language. They are developed to be commercial devices designed to be sold in many countries, and so they are programmed for generic use. In contrast, animals adapt to the cultural identity of the person or family they live with and receive culture-specific attention and training; so, in theory, we may assume they are "culturally appropriate" animals.

The box below provides the summary of key points.

Summary of Key Points

- The cultural iceberg theory
  - Three levels of culture: (1) Visible/conscious; (2) Invisible/subconscious; and (3) Hidden/only known by members of the same cultural group.
- The theory of cultural relativism
  - Universal values are experienced and may be understood differently in different cultures.
  - The importance of understanding cultures in their own terms, without judging them according to external standards.

- It is crucial to understand the background and justification of dangerous cultural practices and be competent and compassionate in the way we communicate disagreement.
- The posthumanist theory and culture
  - Posthumanism seeks to remove the central position occupied by the humans of our planet and aims to expand our understanding of the world by including nonhuman entities such as animals, plants, and machines.

Cultural Identity

Stuart Hall, a prominent cultural theorist, defined cultural identity in 1990 in his essay 'Cultural Identity and Diaspora' as the sense of belonging and attachment that individuals have to a particular cultural or ethnic group. It encompasses the shared beliefs, values, customs, traditions, and language that define a group and distinguish it from others. Cultural identity is often shaped by factors such as ancestry, religion, nationality, and geographic location, among others. According to Hall (1990), cultural identity is not fixed, innate, or pure, but it is multiple and hybrid, constantly changing and evolving over time.

Cultural identity is important for people's sense of self and how they relate to others. It also provides people with access to social networks that provide support and shared values and aspirations. These can help break down barriers and build a sense of trust between people.

Srivastava (2023, p. 59) declared that almost daily all of us negotiate and navigate multiple identities. She provided the following key features about identity:

1. Different identities are prominent under different circumstances.
2. Intersections of identities can significantly influence experience.
3. Identities are often ascribed by others and may have different meanings for others than for the individuals being labelled due to the problematic nature of labels.
4. Cultural identity, like culture, is also dynamic and can shift over time and place.

Understanding and valuing our own cultural identity enable us to recognize and appreciate the diversity of others. This understanding allows us to interact with people from different cultures in a way that is respectful and responsive to their needs. Therefore, cultural identity is a crucial component of developing cultural competence.

The summary of key points is provided in the following box.

Summary of Key Points

- Cultural identity is the sense of belonging and attachment that individuals have to a particular cultural or ethnic group.
- Cultural identity is not fixed, innate, or pure, but it is multiple and hybrid, constantly changing and evolving over time.
- Understanding and valuing our own cultural identity enable us to recognize and appreciate the diversity of others.

The Impact of Culture on Health and Well-being

The impact of culture on health and well-being is not a new concept to be explored. As we discovered at the beginning of this chapter, the search for health and happiness dates back to ancient times. Historical evidence from many civilizations across the world provides many examples. I am providing here three explanations from the ancient Greek history, as I believe that history not only provides information about our past but can also help us shape our future health and well-being.

The 5th century BC was the golden era of Athens. Pericles (495–429 BC)—the leader of the city—promoted the arts, literature, philosophy, and science; it is principally through his efforts that Athens acquired the reputation of being the educational and cultural centre of the ancient Greek world. Pericles also strengthened the democracy in the city and commissioned the building of the Parthenon. Culture and civilization were at their peak, and the Athenian people flourished during this period. However, around 429–426 BC, the 'Plague of Athens' killed almost a quarter of its population, including their leader Pericles.

Hippocrates (460–c.375 BC), an ancient Greek physician and philosopher, believed that good health was not only physical but also psychological and spiritual (Schiefsky, 2005). He argued that culture and civilization were necessary for promoting good health, as they provided opportunities for individuals to develop their intellect, character, and social connections, which are essential for achieving a healthy and fulfilling life (Schiefsky, 2005).

Before I move to current times and explanations, I want to share some Aristotelian wisdom. Aristotle (384–322 BC) was concerned with how an individual should best live their life and asserted the idea that the most virtuous life will be the happiest one. By living well, in balance with one's environment, avoiding excess, and guiding one's life by reason, Aristotle argued, is the path toward the most virtuous and thus the happiest life (Ross & Brown, 2009).

The aforementioned examples clearly indicate the impact of culture on our health and well-being.

As mentioned earlier in this chapter, our 21st- century society faces severe challenges such as mental health crises, an aging population, growing inequalities, forceful displacement of people due to war and political conflict, and huge changes in the workplace due to the fast-developing advanced technologies. The recent report from the European Commission *"Get inspired! Culture: A driver for health and well-being in the EU"* (2022) summarizes the findings of a number of research studies from Erasmus+, Horizon 2020, and Horizon Europe, which deal specifically with the culture and health. One of the included projects is *CultureForHealth* (Zbranca et al., 2022), which throws light on the pathways through which culture and the arts can support individuals and communities to adequately address these global challenges. The report states that good health and well-being are a fundamental pillar of prosperous societies. The *CultureForHealth* research team updated and widened the scope of the WHO (World Health Organization) report *"What is the evidence on the role of the arts in improving health and wellbeing? A scoping review"* (Fancourt & Finn, 2019), which demonstrated that the arts can potentially impact disease prevention and health promotion in the mental and physical health areas, as well as in the management and treatment of illnesses, and found 138 scientific studies regarding the links between culture and health, along with 118 studies on culture and subjective well-being, 131 studies on the culture and community well-being, and 12 studies on culture's positive effects during COVID-19. These studies have enriched the growing body of evidence about the beneficial health and well-being effects of culture.

Most studies conclude that on the societal level, supporting cultural activities in communities could be a key contributor to a holistic health strategy, counterbalancing loneliness and isolation, and, at the same time, promoting health and well-being for all.

However, according to the WHO European Health Equity Status Report Initiative report (2019), 90% of health inequalities can be explained by five factors: quality of healthcare; financial insecurity; poor quality housing and neighborhood environment; social exclusion; and the lack of decent work and poor working conditions. This means that the (WHO, 2019) social determinants of health have a bigger impact on health promotion than individual lifestyle risk factors.

The evidence gathered by the *Culture-ForHealth* research team (Zbranca et al., 2022) suggests that cultural participation can increase knowledge and awareness of various health conditions among underserved communities and provide support networks for disadvantaged individuals suffering from illness.

The WHO report also highlights the significant loss and suffering of forcibly displaced people and their effects on physical and psychological health. Organizing cultural activities for displaced people in their host communities can help support coping and promote recovery and integration, resulting in better health and well-being.

The summary of key points is provided in the box below.

Summary of Key Points

- The search for health and happiness dates back to ancient times.
- Hippocrates argued that culture and civilization were necessary for promoting good health, as they provided opportunities for individuals to develop their intellect, character, and social connections, which are essential for achieving a healthy and fulfilling life.
- Recent reports by the European Commission and the World Health Organization throw light on the pathways through which culture and the arts can support individuals and communities to adequately address the challenges of our century.

Health and Illness

Health refers to a state of well-being that is culturally defined, valued, and practiced and reflects the ability of individuals (or groups) to perform their daily activities in culturally expressed, beneficial, and patterned lifeways (Leininger, 1991). Illness refers to an unwanted condition that is culturally defined and culturally responded to (Papadopoulos, 2006). Western societies may view disease as a result of natural "scientific" phenomena and encourage the use of technology to diagnose and treat disease. Other societies, including indigenous groups, may believe that illness is the result of supernatural phenomena and may promote a range of cultural practices, as well as prayer or other spiritual interventions (McLaughlin & Braun, 1998). Thus, culturally shaped notions of health and illness may have a strong impact on how individuals engage in help seeking and how they view and use the health services (Campbell & Long, 2014).

An immensely necessary component in the formation of the nurse–patient relationship is that of communication. To achieve effective therapeutic communication is challenging, but this can be aided by nurses and other healthcare providers understanding their patients' cultural values, beliefs, and practices. In doing so, healthcare professionals will competently engage with their patient to compare their own health and illness beliefs and values with those of their own, to consider the similarities and differences, and to reach a culturally acceptable and beneficial compromise. This is a most important step toward providing culturally competent and compassionate care that promotes health and alleviates illness.

Culture can have a significant impact on health and well-being. People from different cultural backgrounds may have different beliefs, attitudes, and behaviors related to health, illness, and healthcare. These differences can affect how people understand and respond to health information, how they seek and access healthcare services, and how they make decisions about their health.

Overall, understanding the impact of culture on health and well-being is important in developing effective health promotion and healthcare strategies that take into account the diverse beliefs and practices of different cultural groups.

The box below provides the summary of key point.

Summary of Key Points

- Culturally shaped notions of health and illness may have a strong impact on how individuals engage in help seeking and how they view and use the health services.

- To achieve effective therapeutic communication is challenging, but this can be aided by nurses and other healthcare providers understanding their patients' cultural values, beliefs, and practices.

- Understanding the impact of culture on health and well-being is important in developing effective health promotion and strategies that consider the diverse beliefs and practices of different cultural groups.

Conclusion

In this chapter, we have explored the profound influence that culture exerts on health and well-being. We gained a historical perspective on the concept of culture. We also discovered the fundamental components of key cultural theories and learned how culture develops, evolves, and impacts all aspects of the human experience.

As we examined cultural identity more closely, it became clear that culture is a core part of how individuals see themselves and make sense of the world around them. An individual's cultural affiliations provide a framework for understanding illness, healing practices, family roles, communication styles, and so much more.

We also delved into the various external influences that can shape a culture over time, such as technological advances, globalization, migration patterns, and major historical events. Cultures are not static but continuously adapt and evolve based on these dynamic forces. As cultures shift, it can significantly impact health beliefs, practices, and outcomes within those communities.

Ultimately, this chapter has underscored that culture is an integral part of the human experience—shaping our realities, identities, and paths toward well-being. By continuing to explore culture's profound impact, we can work toward more inclusive, equitable, and effective systems of care for all. Overall, culture is a complex and multifaceted concept that encompasses a wide range of dimensions, each of which can shape the way people think, behave, and interact with one another. Understanding these dimensions is crucial for developing a deeper appreciation and understanding of the diverse cultures that make up our world.

Activities

PERSONAL REFLECTION

Take some time to reflect on your own cultural background, beliefs, and values related to health and healthcare. Consider factors such as family traditions, religious or spiritual beliefs, dietary habits, communication styles, and attitudes toward medical treatments. Write down your thoughts in your diary.

CASE STUDY

Read the following case study and answer the questions that follow:

- Mrs. Chan is a 70-year-old Chinese woman who has been admitted to the hospital because she vomited blood twice during the day. She is accompanied by her son who is also her interpreter.
- What is the best way for the nurse to approach Mrs. Chan in order to conduct her initial assessment?
- What potential cultural factors may be influencing Mrs. Chan's behavior and attitudes toward healthcare?
- What strategies could the nurse employ to promote cultural competence and ensure Mrs. Chan's needs are met?

REFERENCES

Boas, F. (1962). *Anthropology and modern life*. Norton. https://archive.org/details/anthropologymode-00boas.

Braidotti, R. (2013). *The posthuman*. Polity Press.

Campbell, R. D., & Long, L. A. (2014). Culture as a social determinant of mental and behavioral health: A look at culturally shaped beliefs and their impact on help-seeking behaviors and service use patterns of black Americans with depression. *Best Practices in Mental Health: An International Journal, 10*(2), 48–62.

Casanova, J. (2011). Religion, European secular identities, and European integration. *Social Research: An International Quarterly, 78*(4), 1045–1074.

European Commission, Directorate-General for Education, Youth, Sport and Culture. (2022). *Get inspired!—Culture—A driver for health and wellbeing in the EU*. Publications Office of the European Union.

Fancourt, D., & Finn, S. (2019). *What is the evidence on the role of the arts in improving health and wellbeing? A scoping review. Health Evidence Network synthesis report, 67*.

Fernando, S. (1991). *Mental health, race and culture*. Macmillan/Mind Publications.

Friel, S., Marmot, M., Bell, R., Houeling, TAJ., Taylor, S. (2008). WHO Commission on Social Determinants of Health: closing the gap in a generation. Geneva, World Health Organization. https://iris.who.int/bitstream/handle/10665/43943/9789241563703_eng.pdf?sequence=1.

Gandhi, M. K. (1932). *Young India*. Navajivan Trust.

Hall, E. T. (1984). *The dance of life*. Anchor Press.

Hall, S. (1990). Cultural identity and diaspora. In J. Rutherford (Ed.), *Identity: community, culture, difference* (pp. 222–237). Lawrence and Wishart.

Haraway, D. (1985). *Simians, cyborgs and women: the reinvention of nature*. Routledge.

Hassan, I. (1977). Prometheus as performer: toward a post-humanist culture? *The Georgia Review, 31*(4), 830–850.

Kavanagh, H. K., & Kennedy, P. H. (1992). *Promoting cultural diversity*. Sage.

Kenny, A. (2013). *Aristotle poetics. Oxford world's classics*. Oxford University Press.

Legge, J. (Translator). (1971). *Confucian analects; The great learning, and the doctrine of the mean.* Dover Publications.

Leininger, M. M. (1991). *Culture care, diversity and universality: A theory of nursing.* National League for Nursing.

Leininger, M. M. (1995). *Transcultural nursing. Concepts, theories, research, and practices.* McGraw-Hill.

Mandela, N. (1995). *Long walk to freedom.* Abacus.

McLaughlin, L. A., Kathryn, L., & Braun, K. L. (1998). Asian and pacific islander cultural values: Considerations for health care decision making. *Health & Social Work, 23*(2), 116–126. https://doi.org/10.1093/hsw/23.2.116.

Papadopoulos, I., & Koulouglioti, C. (2022). From stories to scenarios and guidelines for the programming of culturally competent, socially assistive robots (Chapter 7, pp.133–164). In I. Papadopoulos, C. Koulouglioti, C. Papadopoulos, & A. Sgorbissa, (Eds.), *Transcultural artificial intelligence and robotics in health and social care.* Elsevier.

Papadopoulos, I. (2006). *Transcultural health and social care: Development of culturally competent practitioners.* Churchill Livingstone Elsevier.

Ritzer, G. (1993). *The McDonaldization of society.* Pine Forge Press.

Ross, W. D. (2009). *Nicomachean ethics.* Contributor. In I. Brown, (Ed) Oxford world's classics. Oxford University Press.

Schiefsky, M. (2005). *Hippocrates on ancient medicine.* Brill.

Schwab, K. (2016). The fourth industrial revolution: What it means, how to respond. *World Economic Forum.* https://www.weforum.org/agenda/2016/01/the-fourth-industrial-revolution-what-it-means-and-how-to-respond/.

Srivastava, R. (2023). *The health care professional's guide to cultural competence* (2nd ed.). Elsevier.

Woodward, S. (2007). The influence of historical events on contemporary culture. *Arts and Humanities in Higher Education, 6*(1), 63–77.

World Health Organization. (WHO). (2019). *The WHO European health equity status report initiative: Case studies.* Retrieved from https://apps.who.int/iris/handle/10665/346050.

Zbranca, R., Dâmaso, M., Blaga, O., Kiss, K., Dascl, M. D., Yakobson, D., & Pop, O. (2022). *Culture-ForHealth Report. Culture's contribution to health and well-being. A report on evidence and policy recommendations for Europe. Culture action Europe.* www.cultureforhealth.eu.

Chapter 2

Cultural Competence for the 21st Century

Learning Objectives

After reading this chapter you should:

- Become aware of the historical aspects of cultural competence.
- Become familiar with essential definitions, theories, and models.
- Gain a detailed knowledge and understanding of the Papadopoulos theory and practice.
- Be introduced to the posthuman theory and its relevance to care.
- Appreciate the relevance of cultural competence in today's world and in the caring professions.
- Familiarize yourself with the E.M.B.R.A.C.E. approach to delivering culturally competent care in the posthuman era.

Introduction

This chapter addresses the need for culturally competent and compassionate care to all patients and clients in the health and care sectors. It reminds the reader that all humans are cultural beings and all societies are multicultural; therefore, it is essential that care must be culturally competent and companionate.

THE GENESIS OF CULTURAL COMPETENCE

Inspired by the American civil rights activist Martin Luther King, Jr. (1929–1968) and his unforgettable "I Have a Dream" speech, during which he called for social change and the end of racism in the United States, I too have a dream! My dream is about radical changes in nursing, particularly transcultural nursing.

Transcultural nursing has been with us for nearly 70 years. The dream of its founder, Dr. Madeleine Leininger (1925–2012), was that the culture care needs of all people will be met by nurses prepared in transcultural nursing. Although during the last 70 years transcultural nursing has developed a huge corpus of knowledge, I can say with some confidence that globally we are far away from Dr. Leininger's dream.

Societies have always included multicultural elements. For example, England has a long and varied history, which resulted from the arrival of people of many cultures and countries in the world, for various reasons. These people brought with them their customs, rituals, religions, cultural beliefs and values, as well as many other cultural elements; many married indigenous residents of England, thus adding a new dimension in the multicultural nature of England. Some of those who arrived in England are:

Romans: AD 43–410

Saxons, Angles, Jutes (Germany/Denmark): 449–700

Vikings (Scandinavia): 800–1066
Normans (France): 1066
West African slaves: 1500–1800
Asians (India): 1600
Huguenots (France): 1670
Russian Jews: 1880
Irish: 1840
Indian soldiers: 1914
German Jews: 1933
Polish/Italians: post-World War II
Commonwealth countries: 1948
Free EU movement: 2004

And the arrival of migrants and refugees of the 21st century.

The genesis of the cultural competence in the 20th century was inevitable. In Chapter 1, the notion of culture and its significance, dating back to ancient times, was discussed. Following the Second World War and the development of the Universal Declaration of Human Rights (UDHR) (United Nations General Assembly, 1948), governments, international organizations, and the public became more aware and sensitized to the human violations perpetrated on the public and especially the vulnerable people by the privileged, the powerful, the greedy, the immoral, and the criminal sections of societies.

The UDHR consists of 30 articles, which outline the fundamental rights and freedoms that are inherent to all human beings, regardless of their race, nationality, religion, gender, or any other status. The preamble of the UDHR declares that the recognition of the inherent dignity and equal and inalienable rights of all members of the human family is the foundation of freedom, justice, and peace in the world. Box 2.1 provides some of the articles of the

BOX 2.1 SELECTED UDHR ARTICLES

- All human beings are born free and equal in dignity and rights.
- Everyone is entitled to all the rights and freedoms set forth in this Declaration, without distinction of any kind, such as race, color, sex, language, religion, political or other opinion, national or social origin, property, birth, or other status.
- Everyone has the right to life, liberty, and security of person.
- No one shall be subjected to torture or to cruel, inhuman, or degrading treatment or punishment.
- Everyone has the right to seek and to enjoy in other countries asylum from persecution.
- Everyone has the right to freedom of thought, conscience, and religion.

declaration that are inextricably linked to transcultural health/nursing and cultural competence. Although cultural competence in health and care practice is underpinned by the universal human rights (Papadopoulos, 2006), its approach to care services and practices highlights and promotes the culture-specific manifestations of the UDHR universal principles, as they are enacted in diverse groups. For example, the expression of dignity may differ from culture to culture; how dignity is assured and the level of its assurance will, most likely, also differ. Cultural competence promotes the symbiotic existence of both universal and culture-specific knowledge and practice.

Here are some other milestones in the genesis of cultural competence. Terry L. Cross and his colleagues (1989) are credited with popularizing the term *cultural competence*. The actual term was first used in the field of social work by Derald Wing Sue and colleagues in their 1978 book, *Counselling the*

Culturally Diverse: Theory and Practice (Sue & Sue, 2016).

The concept of cultural competence had been discussed and developed prior and after that time. In nursing, Madeleine Leininger developed the concept of transcultural nursing in the 1950s that emphasized the importance of understanding cultural differences and incorporating cultural beliefs and practices into nursing care. The anthropologist Edward T. Hall discussed the importance of understanding cultural differences in communication in his 1959 book, *The Silent Language*. Milton J. Bennett (1986) developed the much-used Developmental Model of Intercultural Sensitivity (DMIS) in the 1980s. Additionally, the US National Centre for Cultural Competence was established in 1986 to promote the integration of cultural competence in health and human services. The National CLAS Standards (Culturally and Linguistically Appropriate Services) were developed in 2000 by the US Department of Health and Human Services to promote cultural and linguistic competency in health and social services and were first introduced in 2013 (Office of Minority Health, 2013).

I must also mention the social psychologist Geert Hofstede (1928–2020), known for his research on the cultural dimensions of values and beliefs published in his book *Culture's Consequences* (Hofstede, 1980). There are numerous other scholars who have greatly contributed in the development and uptake of the notion of cultural competence.

We must remember that all humans are cultural beings and generally want and deserve to have their cultural identities respected, especially during vulnerable times such as when going through illness, bereavement, major health and natural disasters, wars, and displacement, to name but a few. Cultural identity is considered a human right. The recent wars and conflicts in the Middle and Far East, as well as Ukraine, are adding to the multicultural mix of many countries, thus creating super-diverse societies. It is inevitable that the indigenous and migrant people will need health and social care at some point. There is a huge corpus of evidence that has established the fact that effective, efficient, and compassionate care cannot be achieved unless the workforce is culturally competent. Unfortunately, the health and care services, although subscribing to the importance of culturally competent care, regularly fail to provide the training, leadership, and organizational culture needed to achieve culturally competent care.

But there are other reasons as to why transcultural nursing and cultural competence remain—in many cases—an unfulfilled dream rather than a reality. To begin with, let me declare that classic transcultural nursing theories will always be useful. But the world is changing fast, and, as mentioned already, cultures are becoming more complex and multilayered, and new theories are emerging from other disciplines that provide a different but nevertheless relevant perspectives on humans, on how global health can be addressed, on the new skills needed, and on the importance of multidisciplinary collaborative working. There is an urgency in our transcultural project. This is why the evolution that has been happening in the last 70 years is not enough. This is why we need a revolution.

Essential Definitions, Theories, and Models

DEFINITIONS

Transcultural nursing: Transcultural nursing is a substantive area of study and practice focused on comparative cultural care (caring) values, beliefs, and practices of individuals or groups of similar or different cultures with the goal of providing culture-specific and universal nursing care practices in promoting health or well-being or to help people face unfavorable human conditions, illness, or death in culturally meaningful ways (Leininger, 1995).

Competence is a key aspect of professional practice in the health and care sectors. It is often defined in terms of the knowledge, skills, and attitudes that are necessary to perform a specific role or tasks, effectively and safely, thus providing high-quality care and support to patients and clients. Competence is a key component of professionalism, the values of which underpin their ethical practice, confidentiality, and respect for the patients' rights and autonomy.

Cultural competence expands the aforementioned definition by adding some specific elements. For example, Spector (2017) defined cultural competence as the ability to see patients as unique individuals with their own beliefs, values, and traditions and to provide care that respects and honours those differences.

I have defined cultural competence as the capacity to provide effective and compassionate healthcare taking into consideration people's cultural beliefs, behaviors, and needs. Cultural competence is not an end in itself, but a means to an end. The end is to improve health outcomes for patients and communities, reduce health inequalities, and promote social justice. Cultural competence is an ongoing process of learning, reflection, and self-awareness. It requires nurses (and other health and care workers) to constantly examine their own cultural assumptions and biases and to engage in a process of life-long learning and professional development (Papadopoulos, 2006).

Key concepts associated with cultural competence are culture, multiculturalism, ethnicity, race, diversity, racism, prejudice, and oppression. I have discussed the problematic nature of defining these concepts and provided my chosen definitions and explanations of them in Chapter 1.

Although cultural competence in nursing was originally viewed as the vehicle to deliver the transcultural nursing theory, it gradually evolved to produce a number of conceptual models with their unique theoretical underpinnings.

However, the term *cultural competence*, and its perception of what it means, is not universally accepted. In 1998, Melanie Tervalon and Jann Murray-Garcia criticized cultural competence in their article, "Cultural Humility Versus Cultural Competence: A Critical Distinction in Defining Physician Training Outcomes in Multicultural Education." The key criticisms included the essentializing of cultures due to simplification and generalization of diverse cultures by failing to recognize their complexity. They also argued that cultural competence reinforces power imbalance between health services and marginalized communities, forcing them to adapt to the dominant culture. According to them, cultural competence focuses on knowledge without addressing the underlying factors influencing care. Instead of cultural competence, they proposed the 'cultural humility' approach, which they defined as a lifelong commitment to self-evaluation and critique in order to redress the power imbalances in the patient–healthcare professionals' dynamic and to develop mutually beneficial partnerships with communities and defined populations.

Another critique to cultural competence originated by Earley and Soon Ang in their 2003 book, *Cultural Intelligence: Individual Interactions Across Cultures*. The term *cultural intelligence* was defined as the ability to adapt to new cultural contexts and work effectively in situations characterized by cultural diversity. They argue that cultural intelligence is essential for success in today's globalized world, where people from different cultures frequently interact in business, education, and other fields. In their 2008 *Handbook of Cultural Intelligence*, Ang and Van Dyne refer to the work of Gelfand et al. (2008), "Thinking Intelligently About Cultural Intelligence: The Road Ahead," who provided a critical comment regarding the limitations of cultural competence. They stated that despite years of scholarship across multiple disciplines, progress in understanding cultural competencies has been limited theoretically, methodologically, and practically.

The literature can perhaps be characterized as suffering from the jingle and jangle fallacy (Kelley, 1927), where constructs with the same meaning are labeled differently while constructs with different meanings are labeled similarly. For example, terms such as both *cultural sensitivity and cultural empathy* refer to an ability to empathize with the feelings, thoughts, and behaviors of people from different cultures (Van Oudenhoven & Van der Zee, 2002). It was also suggested that there is much confusion and misunderstanding about what exactly cultural competence entails, with no overarching theoretical framework to tie the numerous constructs together and little consensus regarding the operationalization of cultural competence. The critics conclude that in such confusion, the practical utility of cultural competencies is undoubtedly compromised.

The main common criticism of the originators of both cultural intelligence and cultural humility is that cultural competence emphasizes the acquisition of knowledge about different cultures without necessarily emphasizing the importance of building relationships with people from those cultures and being willing to learn from them. These and other criticisms can be challenged in many ways, one of which is by reading the comprehensive work published by healthcare academics and practitioners. Nevertheless, both cultural intelligence and cultural humility enrich the field by providing different frameworks, which may be preferred by some who work in the health and social care sectors. Furthermore, we should reflect on the criticisms and address any evidenced comments. I believe that despite their differences, all these models and theories aim to achieve similar outcomes: to reduce health inequalities and promote flexible, sensitive, and appropriate care to patients, families, and the public.

THEORIES AND MODELS

Most people agree that a theory is a well-supported and tested explanation of a phenomenon that can be used to make predictions and guide future research. Theories are typically highly specific, incorporating a set of interconnected concepts and principles that explain a particular aspect of the world.

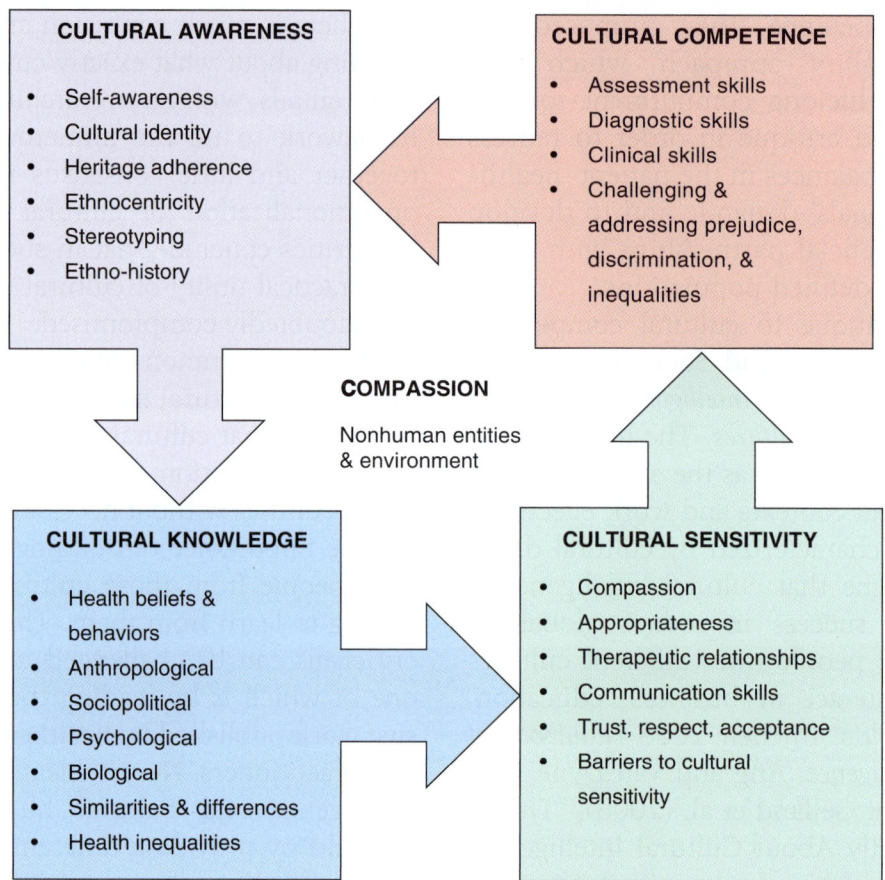

Figure 2.1 The Papadopoulos model of cultural competence (2006, 2018). (Modified from Papadopoulos, I., Shea, S., Taylor, G. et al. (2016). Developing tools to promote culturally competent compassion, courage, and intercultural communication in healthcare. *Journal of Compassionate Health Care, 3*(2). https://doi.org/10.1186/s40639-016-0019-6)

A conceptual model is a simplified representation of a complex system or phenomenon that is used to help understand and explain it. Conceptual models are usually represented as diagrams. Conceptual models are often used to illustrate relationships between different elements or to demonstrate how a process works.

In 1998, myself and two colleagues—Dr. Mary Tilki and Dr. Gina Taylor—published the book, *Transcultural Care: A Guide for Health Care Professionals*, which included the Papadopoulos, Tilki, and Taylor model of cultural competence (Papadopoulos et al., 1998). The

model was developed during a research project we undertook in the early 1990s among nurse teachers. In the 1998 book, limited information was published about the model's underpinned values and principles and about the model's emerging theory. In 2006, I revised the model and provided all the missing theoretical elements in my book, *Transcultural Health and Social Care: Development of Culturally Competent Practitioners*.

As you can see in Figure 2.1, the model consists of four key constructs: Cultural Awareness, Cultural Knowledge, Cultural Sensitivity, and Cultural Competence. A conceptual map is provided for each construct as a guideline only. Educators may add other concepts or modify the proposed ones to suit the type and level of students.

In the centre of the model, the concept of compassion is placed. I believe that compassion is the essence of nursing and healthcare in general. Compassion permeates all the four domains of this model as it involves recognizing and responding to the unique needs and suffering of others, with kindness, understanding, and empathy. A new addition to the model is the posthuman notions and links to nonhuman entities and the environment, which I briefly discussed in Chapter 1. This new component to the model will be further discuss in Chapter 3.

I conducted two international studies on compassion in nursing (Papadopoulos et al., 2017, 2020), which revealed the cultural components and actions of conscious and intentional compassion. The components were time, being there, going the extra mile, defending, advocating, and personalizing. Some of the associated actions were active listening, developing therapeutic relationships, sharing common humanity, challenging stereotypes, injustices, and discrimination, as well as promoting equality, acknowledging the uniqueness of individuals and their needs, all of which strengthen the foundations of nursing, in particular transcultural nursing, and the engine of the vehicle which delivers it, that of cultural competence.

The revised model (Papadopoulos, 2006) is underpinned by the following pillars:

a Values:
- Human rights
- Compassion
- Courage
- Social justice
- Practical wisdom

b Principles:
- Sociopolitical systems
- Intercultural education
- World citizenship
- National and international law

CASE STUDY: MRS. AHMET

Let us now walk through the four key constructs of the Papadopoulos model of cultural competence using a scenario involving Mrs. Ahmet and her family.

Mrs. Ahmet is a 70-year-old Muslim woman who arrived from Pakistan 5 years ago to stay with her only son who has been living in England with his wife and two children for the last 15 years. Mrs. Ahmet does not speak English. Just over a year ago, she noticed a lump on her breast but did not say anything to her son or daughter-in-law, as she was embarrassed and also did not want to bother them. They both work full time and often leave home early in the morning and return late and very tired. Being a faithful Muslim, Mrs. Ahmet believes that Allah can heal diseases, so she reads the Quran and prays five times a day. Lately, her family noticed that she was losing weight and often complained of fatigue as well as aches and pains. She is now in hospital and has been diagnosed with advanced-stage breast cancer and secondary deposits in her lungs.

The team who is looking after Mrs. Ahmet includes an English specialist nurse, a Polish nurse and a Nigerian nurse, an English male oncology consultant, a Bulgarian female junior doctor, a Filipina healthcare assistant, and an Indian healthcare assistant.

Mrs. Ahmet's son informed the nurses that he does not wish them to tell his mother about her diagnosis. He wants to protect her from all the stress and sadness she will have if she knew her diagnosis. He also wishes his mother to be given all available treatments in order to arrest the cancer and give her the best chance for prolonging her life. He does not see the need for a professional interpreter, as he has taken time off work, and he and his wife and teenage children can be available to act as translators.

Cultural Awareness

The first stage in the model is cultural awareness, which begins with an exploration of our personal values and beliefs, our cultural identity, heritage, ethnohistory, and so on. Self-awareness is based on the Socratic dictum of 'know thyself' (aftognosia), which is the path to a virtuous life that guides our actions toward understanding, caring, and respecting ourselves. As our self is not complete without a relationship with another self, we need to reflect and become aware of the importance of learning and understanding the other person's cultural identity in order to avoid stereotyping them or treating them inappropriately (Box 2.2).

BOX 2.2 ACTIVITY: CULTURAL AWARENESS REFLECTIONS

- We need to ask ourselves and reflect on some relevant questions, such as:
  - Am I aware of my own worldview and what influenced and shaped it?
  - How do my cultural values and upbringing impact on the way I treat others?
  - Do I judge those in my care before I have enough information about the cultural identity and heritage?
  - Am I ethnocentric and how does this impact on those in my care?

So, how does the notion of cultural awareness help provide appropriate care to Mrs. Ahmet?

Spending a little time thinking about our own cultural background will make us realize what values we hold and why. Hopefully, we will discover values, attitudes, and beliefs that are hidden deep in our subconsciousness but that could surface when we are stressed and demonstrate that, like all human beings, we too can stereotype and be ethnocentric. This self-reflection will help us prepare to deal with such events when they happen.

Spending time to find out where Mrs. Ahmet comes from, why she left her country, and what values she holds will make us realize that even though all human beings have much in common, our small or subtle differences are important, as they are the ones that define our uniqueness and our cultural identity.

An obvious difference between Mrs. Ahmet and the nurses is likely to be their religion. As an older woman, she may still hold the view that as a patient she must unquestionably listen to and do what the doctors and nurses tell her to do. She is very likely to accept her son's judgments. The nurses and doctors may find her passive role less accepting, as they have been socialized to believe that it is best to be actively involved in our care. Not being able to communicate directly with her due to language issues makes it less likely to challenge our stereotypes about Mrs. Ahmet.

Cultural Knowledge

The next key construct of the model is cultural knowledge, which can be gained in a number of ways such as meaningful contact with ordinary people from different cultural groups. This can enhance our knowledge around their health beliefs and behaviors as well as raise our understanding around the health and social challenges and problems they may be facing.

Learning from our patients is also a way to gain knowledge, and this is based on the belief that culture is individually and socially constructed rather than being a static entity. However, this approach is not always possible, as, for example, when a patient is unconscious or extremely ill or as in the case of Mrs. Ahmet who does not speak English. We should of course use an interpreter—in her case members of her family—but this may only partly be helpful. Even if the caring team could use a professional interpreter for Mrs. Ahmet, access to them must be organized, which may take time. In the 21st century, care staff have access to smart voice-activated audio devices, which can help with translation, as well as computers, which enable the care team to write information or questions in the language of the patient who then replies in her/his language. However, some older migrants—such as in the case of Mrs. Ahmet—may be illiterate, and such approaches are inappropriate. The kind of learning the care staff need to acquire about their patients often happens over the period of time during assessments and the provision of care as well as during naturally occurring contacts with her. The problem with using our patients to educate us is that some patients may see this as a burden and may not be willing to do so. Irrespective of the approach we use to gain cultural knowledge, it is advisable to have some culture-generic information about health beliefs, customs, religious rituals, diet, hygiene practices, maintenance of privacy and dignity, etc., about a range of patients we most frequently encounter.

Health inequalities is something the Papadopoulos, Tilki, and Taylor model gives serious attention to. This is because even though all human beings are cultural beings and therefore their cultural beliefs and behaviors should be taken into consideration, we all know that health inequalities are far more extensive in people from minority ethnic groups, who do worse than the indigenous population in almost all health indicators. It would be convenient to blame the health problems experienced by these people on their culture. Sadly, some politicians and even health professionals do. But the evidence that has been amassed in the last 20–30 years (e.g., WHO, 2008, 2019) points to the fact that these health inequalities are linked to other structural inequalities and discrimination experienced by people from minority ethnic groups, such as poor housing, unemployment, lack of educational opportunities, social exclusion, as well as inaccessible health services. It is for this reason that this model is probably the only model that explicitly has, over the years, put equal emphasis on both culture and structure (Box 2.3).

BOX 2.3 ACTIVITY: CULTURAL KNOWLEDGE REFLECTIONS

- Do I know enough about the cultural beliefs and values of those in my care, such as Mrs. Ahmet?
  - How do my different values and beliefs impact on those in my care for Mrs. Ahmet?
  - Do I use the power I have as a healthcare professional to advocate and promote the reduction of health inequalities?

Cultural Sensitivity

An important element in achieving cultural sensitivity is how professionals view people in their care. Unless clients/patients are considered true partners, culturally sensitive care is not being achieved. If we do not consider them true partners, we risk using our professional power in an oppressive way. Equal partnerships, according to this model, involve trust, acceptance, and respect, as well as facilitation and negotiation.

A key factor in achieving the elements of cultural sensitivity is learning to ask the right questions. Having the necessary awareness and culture-generic knowledge will enable us to anticipate needs and ask questions with the right content, thus minimizing the risk of misunderstandings. But achieving the levels of interpersonal communication needed to establish a trusting and therapeutic relationship requires compassion.

Aristotle (384–322 BCE) reminds us that compassion is the ability to recognize the suffering of others and to allow others to know that we really care (Aristotle, 2004). Are we born compassionate? Of course not, but Aristotle again assures us that humans can learn and cultivate the virtue of compassion and of course other virtues such as courage. He taught that virtues are like habits that are practiced and strengthened with use. A culturally competent health professional is one who possesses—always according to Aristotle—the virtue of courage to challenge accepted norms and practices that harm, discriminate, or disadvantage people in our care.

All patients are vulnerable when they are receiving treatment as outpatient or at home. But they are more so when they are admitted to the hospital. Cultural sensitivity and all the elements and skills we discussed so far should enable us to develop a therapeutic relationship with Mrs. Ahmet. Is there anything else that a nurse should consider in order to form this relationship and help Mrs. Ahmet?

Some of the challenges for Mrs. Ahmet and the caring team may be as follows:

- Limited acculturation: She has not been in England long enough to acculturate, and she probably spent most of her time at home looking after the family.
- Communication: Her inability to speak English is probably causing her a lot of anxiety.
- Limited familiarity with the English healthcare system: Due to this limitation, she lacks the confidence to act independently. She is frightened being in a strange environment.
- Values and religion: Her cultural values and religious beliefs will differ from most of the members of the healthcare team and she worries whether they understand them.
- She worries in case the staff will not like her because she is a migrant and may ignore her because she cannot communicate with them.

But there are challenges within the healthcare team too, such as their own differences in cultural and religious values; the understanding of each team member of the professional hierarchies and gender differences within the team; their own professional and life experiences, especially for those members who have not been in England for long and had completed their professional studies in their countries of origin; the fact that Mrs. Ahmet is an elderly woman with advanced cancer; her son's requests, which most likely go against their professional codes of conduct; and so on.

Cultural sensitivity requires that the healthcare team looking after Mrs. Ahmet need to show her that they recognize her pain and anxiety and that they care. They do not need to speak the same language to be able to do this. A gentle smile, acknowledging her presence, or a greeting in Urdu will make her feel wanted and cared for.

The healthcare team will respect the request of her family to act as interpreters, but they will equally state that since the family members will not be at her bedside for 24 hours a day, they may need to seek the assistance of a professional interpreter. An interpreter will provide her with information about the care and medical procedures she will receive and inform her that they will supply food acceptable to her and support her religious needs. Above all, the caring team need to recognize that her family members are very important to her and allow her to see them without too many restrictions in time and numbers.

Involving her family in her care and decision-making is also important. She will expect this. Finding a way to negotiate the differences between her son's views and the healthcare team's views is another priority that must be handled sensitively. The care team must try to understand why her son feels the way he does and explain their reasons for having different views. Patients and family members could have stereotypes about health professionals and health services. They have probably heard stories from their friends who may have had negative experiences, and they fear this may happen to them. They have suspicions about things they do not understand and have not had explained to them. However, with sensitivity and patience, most people find solutions and reach compromises.

Cultural Competence

The achievement of cultural competence requires the synthesis and application of previously gained awareness, knowledge, and sensitivity. Emphasis is given to practical skills such as assessment of needs, clinical diagnosis, and other caring skills. An important component in this last key construct of the model is the ability to recognize and challenge racism and other forms of discrimination and oppressive practice (Box 2.4).

But as we noted earlier, the act of challenging requires courage. However, courage without wisdom is dangerous for both the person who is committing the unwise courageous act and the persons for whom it is committed. Gaining the practical wisdom to recognize unfairness and to challenge it effectively is a virtue we must learn to use. This will be discussed in more detail in Chapter 3.

BOX 2.4 ACTIVITY: CULTURAL COMPETENCE REFLECTIONS

- Some relevant questions to reflect on are as follows:
  - Am I competently applying my cultural awareness, knowledge, and sensitivity in my practice?
  - Am I courageous enough to speak up and challenge injustice and human rights violations when I see them?
  - Do I possess the practical wisdom to challenge constructively at the right time and through the right channels?
  - Am I aware of the crises facing humankind and do I think about my contributions to relevant solutions?

A good way to assess and plan culturally competent care for Mrs. Ahmet is by following the principles in LEARN as proposed by Berlin and Fowkes in 1982.

LEARN model, which stands for:

L… 'listen' to her perception of her problem;

E… 'explain' your perception of the problem;

A…'acknowledge' the similarities and differences between the two;

R…'recommend' solutions which must involve Mrs. Ahmet and her family;

N…'negotiate' the treatment plan which incorporates relevant aspects of Mrs. Ahmet's culture.

The Relevance of Cultural Competence in Today's World and in the Care Professions

Let us now move to the current health challenges and priorities that urgently need new ways of delivering culturally competent care.

I am sure you will agree that the 21st century has ushered in a technological revolution, not only huge migration waves, environmental disasters, global conflicts and terrorism, global economic crises, and pandemic disasters with millions of people dying (e.g., COVID-19) but also huge advances in medical sciences, resulting in the extension of life and the increase in the numbers of very old people and centenarians. Almost all this century's challenges listed are human made. It is time to search for new perspectives and adopt new approaches and solutions.

In my view, society, including nursing and other care services, is entering the posthumanist era, described as a philosophical and cultural movement that emerged in the late 20th century and which challenges traditional notions of what it means to be human. It is characterized by a rejection of human exceptionalism and a belief that humans are not the only beings with agency, consciousness, moral code, or intelligence. This is a new theory that deserves our attention.

In her article, "Existential Posthumanism: A Manifesto," Francesca Ferrando (2023), one of the most prominent proponents of posthumanism, explains that existential posthumanism was the result of the existential crisis and awakenings generated by the COVID-19 pandemic. She states that there is no need to wait for hyper technological futures to be posthuman. We can actually become posthuman right now. For instance, in the ways we, the human species as a whole, live; in the modes we, as individuals, behave; in the forms we, as organisms, interact with the personal, the social, the environmental, the biological, the planetary, the ontological, and beyond. Existential posthumanism as a philosophy of life approaches humans in all of their diversities, nonhuman animals, technological entities, and ecological systems. It deconstructs any discrimination based on human-indexed classification; in other words, the human supremacy in the hierarchy of human and nonhuman entities.

Think about it. Why do we still believe that animals have no feelings, have inferior intelligence than humans, have no consciousness, and are on the planet to be exploited by humans? Some of you may have a pet dog or cat in your house. Have you ever witnessed an animal giving birth and were amazed by the care they take of their offspring? Have you ever seen animals protecting their offspring and moaning over a dead one? Have you ever watched any videos showing a dog giving care to a disabled person or a horse visiting a hospital to provide a few minutes of happiness to a sick child? Have you seen monkeys grooming each other or performing the most intelligent actions when searching for food? Have you ever considered the intelligence and work ethic of a bee? I could go on and on giving examples, but I am sure you understand my point that animals deserve our respect and we can learn valuable life lessons from them.

And what about the crucial role of the environment? Trees and other plants contribute to our survival by providing food and medicines, by cleaning the atmosphere, and by helping stabilize the planet's temperature, thus avoiding even more natural disasters.

Why am I talking about nature and the planet? Because they are fundamental building blocks in the creation and shaping of cultures. By understanding the impact of nature and the geology of our planet, we will most likely gain a deeper appreciation of our roots, respect our cultural differences, eliminate— or at least reduce—discrimination toward humans and nonhuman entities, explore our connectedness, and preserve the balance of the planet, realizing that humans, the fauna and flora of our planet, and the coming of intelligent robots are equally important to life. These relationships should be acknowledged in any understanding of what it means to be human. It is therefore crucial that nursing embraces the posthuman philosophy to bring about the nursing revolution we need to have (Box 2.5).

Let us now move on to talk about robots and Artificial Intelligence (AI) technologies in the posthuman era. Recently, I was involved in a Horizon 2020 project called CARESSES. The aim of that study was to develop the first socially assistive and culturally competent

BOX 2.5 ENTER POSTHUMANISM

- Posthumanist is described as a philosophical and cultural movement that emerged in the late 20th century.
- Posthumanism challenges traditional notions of what it means to be human. It is characterized by a rejection of human exceptionalism and a belief that humans are not the only beings with agency, consciousness, moral code, or intelligence.
- Posthumanism as a philosophy of life approaches humans in all of their diversities, nonhuman animals, technological entities, and ecological systems.
- It deconstructs any discrimination based on human-indexed classification—in other words, the human supremacy in the hierarchy of human and nonhuman entities.

robot for the care of older people. This was achieved, and it has opened the way for the creation of more socially assistive robots and other AI devices that gradually are being integrated into the everyday work of nurses. The types of these robots vary from helping lift and move patients, to telemedicine robots that facilitate remote consultations, to companion robots, etc.

The COVID-19 pandemic highlighted the possibilities and roles that robots and AI devices can play in the posthuman world and reshape human existence. During the pandemic, many people, including of course those working in health and care services, turned to technology to stay connected with loved ones, work remotely, access healthcare services, and using telemedicine to consult with doctors.

One of the findings of a research project I conducted in 2021 (Papadopoulos et al., 2022) to explore the provision of spiritual care to hospitalized COVID-19 patients was the reliance of AI devices used by hospital chaplains to deliver spiritual support and religious rituals virtually to patients and their loved ones. It became evident that AI technologies have a major role to play during existential crises such as pandemics and natural disasters like the recent massive earthquake in Turkey and Syria in 2023, as well as in Morocco that same year.

The E.M.B.R.A.C.E. Approach to Delivering Culturally Competent Care in the Posthuman Era

Having discussed in detail the concepts, values, principles, and content of the four key constructs of the Papadopoulos model, I will now try to compare these with those of posthumanism. In order to achieve this, I have organized their components using the acronym **E.M.B.R.A.C.E** (Empathy, Multiculturalism, Bias, Respect, Awareness, Communication, Education).

a *First let me explain what the acronym E.M.B.R.A.C.E stands from the **cultural competence** lens.*

Empathy/Compassion: Cultural competence in health and care require empathy and compassion toward patients of diverse cultural backgrounds, as well as understanding and respecting their values, beliefs, and practices.

Multiculturalism: It is important to acknowledge and embrace the diversity of cultures in health and care settings to provide culturally responsive and appropriate care.

Bias: To provide culturally competent care, healthcare professionals must be aware of their own biases and prejudices and take steps to address them.

Respect: Cultural competence in health and care requires showing respect to patients' cultural beliefs, practices, and values, even if they differ from the healthcare provider's own beliefs.

Awareness: Healthcare providers must be aware of the cultural differences and challenges that patients from different cultural backgrounds may face when accessing health and care services.

Communication: Effective communication is key to providing culturally competent care, and healthcare providers should use appropriate communication styles and techniques that are respectful of patients' cultural backgrounds.

Education: Health and care professionals should engage in ongoing education and training to continually improve their cultural competence and provide the best possible care to patients from diverse cultural backgrounds.

b. *Now let us examine the meaning of acronym E.M.B.R.A.C.E from the posthumanist lens.*

Evolutionary Progression: Posthumanism acknowledges that the evolution of humanity has not ended and that there is a possibility for continued progression into a new form of being.

Machine Learning: As machines become more advanced, posthumanists explore the possibilities of merging human and machine intelligence to create a new type of being.

Bioengineering: Posthumanists are interested in the use of biotechnology to enhance human abilities and extend the human life span.

Robotics: The development of advanced robotics and AI is a key area of interest for posthumanists.

Alternative Reality: Posthumanism explores the possibility of creating alternative realities that are beyond our current understanding of existence.

Cybernetics: Posthumanists are interested in the integration of technology and biology, creating a hybrid being that is both human and machine.

Ethics: Posthumanists are concerned with the ethical implications of creating a new type of being and explore how society should deal with these new ethical issues.

E.M.B.R.A.C.E INTERSECTORS AND CONCILLIATORS

Some of the two sets of the E.M.B.R.A.C.E concepts/components clearly **intersect** with each other while the remaining concepts function as **conciliators**, acting as mediators between cultural competence and posthumanism in order to create collaborations and enable changes to be made on a conceptual continuum with zero change on the one end, evolution in the middle, and revolution at the other end.

a *Intersectors*

Empathy/Compassion: Both cultural competence in health and care and posthumanism emphasize the importance of empathy toward individuals who may be different from oneself. In cultural competence, empathy is used to better understand and accommodate patients from different cultural backgrounds. In posthumanism, empathy

is used to envision and design technologies that enhance or augment human abilities while also consider the needs and desires of posthuman beings.

Multiculturalism: Both cultural competence in health and care and posthumanism acknowledge the existence and importance of diversity. In cultural competence, healthcare providers are encouraged to recognize and respect the cultural backgrounds of their patients. In posthumanism, technological advancements are endeavoring to be inclusive in terms of diversity and cultural competence or appropriateness in order to be acceptable and effective.

Ethics: Both cultural competence and posthumanism grapple with ethical questions related to how individuals should be treated. For example, in cultural competence, ethical considerations involve respecting patients' cultural beliefs and values as well as ensuring that they receive equitable care. In posthumanism, ethical considerations involve questions related to the creation and treatment of posthuman beings, including their rights and autonomy.

b. *Conciliators*

Evolutionary progression: In order to enable the evolutionary progression of humans and other sentient beings, societies should recognize that the current anthropocentric education of people (including that of health and social care professionals) must take on board the posthuman theories. In the 21st century, we have experienced the growing integration of machine learning.

Alternative reality: The introduction of virtual reality is gradually becoming more acceptable in many walks of life, including the education of health professionals. It is inevitable that this technology will continue to advance to create alternative realities that are beyond our current understanding of existence. However, in order to succeed in the field of healthcare, it is imperative that developers are aware of the cultural differences and challenges that patients from different cultural backgrounds may face when accessing health and care services.

Bioengineering: Posthumanists are interested in the use of biotechnology to enhance human abilities and extend the human life span.

Cybernetics: Posthumanists are interested in the integration of technology and biology, creating a hybrid being that is both human and machine.

Communication: Effective communication is key to providing culturally competent care, and healthcare providers should use appropriate communication styles and techniques that are respectful of patients' cultural backgrounds.

Robotics: The development of advanced robotics and AI is a key area of interest for posthumanists.

Respect: Cultural competence in health and care requires showing respect to patients' cultural beliefs, practices, and values, even if they differ from the healthcare provider's own beliefs.

Bias: To provide culturally competent care, healthcare professionals must be aware of their own biases and prejudices and take steps to address them.

Figure 2.2 illustrates the two lenses, cultural competence and posthumanism, each

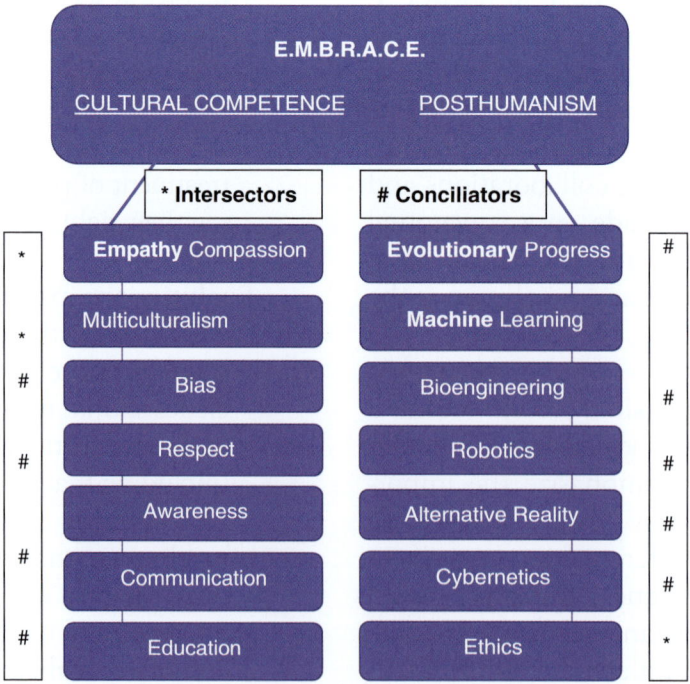

Figure 2.2 The E.M.B.R.A.C.E. approach for delivering culturally competent care in the posthuman era.

with their respective components aligned under the umbrella of E.M.B.R.A.C.E. This visually represents how the concept is approached from both perspectives and how they intersect and interact with each other.

Let me provide some examples of this cultural competence/posthumanism collaboration that may stimulate the revolution we are trying to achieve in order to bring significant changes to transcultural nursing and nursing in general. I recommend that by the end of this decade, nursing should and could change in a number of ways.

Example 1:
The increased use of technology will play a significant role in nursing. Nurses may use more advanced and smart equipment to monitor patient health, input data in electronic health records, conduct telehealth assessments and therapies, etc.

Example 2:
More emphasis on diversity and cultural competence and compassion will continue to be embedded in all aspects of nursing and nursing education.

Example 3:
Virtual reality and AI simulations and virtual reality for the training and educating nursing students will be greatly increased.

Example 4:
As the public becomes more informed and sensitized to their human rights and the laws of their countries, they will expect to receive nondiscriminatory care that is compassionate and culturally competent. It is more likely that more members of the public will sue the care providers if they perceive that their care was inadequate, unsafe, unequal, and disrespectful of their cultural identity and needs.

Example 5:
As healthcare becomes more complex, there will be a growing need for specialist nurses working in collaboration with other professionals who can provide culturally competent care in specific areas such as major health disasters and emergencies and advance technological nursing to populations with no access to a nearby hospital.

Example 6:
With an aging population and a rise in chronic diseases as well as pandemics, a greater emphasis on preventative care in nursing will be in place, which means the provision of culturally appropriate education and the development of culturally effective interactive resources to help patients maintain healthy lifestyles and prevent illness.

Example 7:
The principles of cultural competence and compassion should be included in all nursing and healthcare curricula.

Example 8:
All nursing and healthcare curricula should include the principles of existential posthuman philosophy and its relevance to transcultural nursing.

Example 9:
All health and care teachers should attend a short course on posthumanism to enable them to teach this new theory to their students.

Example 10:
Teaching the knowledge contents of nursing curricula should include fewer classroom sessions and more online learning.

Example 11:
More face-to-face discussions and debates must be included in order to allow the students to reflect on their cultural identities, heritage, ethnohistory, and ethnocentricity, thus raising their levels of self-awareness.

Example 12:
Face-to-face sessions for students should be provided in order to discuss the impact and importance of culture while dispelling the myths and misconceptions of cultures.

Example 13:
Students should be encouraged to engage in collaborative projects to problem-solve scenarios or AI simulations of posthumanist topics such as the interconnectedness of humans, the environment, the nonhuman entities, and other relevant topics.

Example 14:
More emphasis should be given to care skills development such as culturally competent and compassionate communication, culturally appropriate trust, dealing with culture-related conflict, and addressing racism, exclusion, and inequalities by using virtual reality, gamifications, and simulation.

Example 15:
Nurses must be supported or take the initiative in identifying culturally competent technological nursing solutions and submitting their ideas to tech companies or applying for research funding.

Example 16:
By the end of this decade, transcultural nursing education will develop nurses who will possess both theoretical and practical wisdom, thus empowering them to deal better with new and global challenges and make a real difference in the world.

The aforementioned examples highlight a number of challenges that justify my belief that the existing transcultural nursing needs to be revolutionized and changed, and this should start happening not in 5 years or even in 1 year, but now.

Conclusion

This chapter provided a number of themes that help the reader understand the origins and importance of cultural competence in health and care sectors. The chapter also presented current and future theories and models, in the hope that they will stimulate needed changes in organizational and individual care planning and interventions. Practical examples and recommendations have been given to enable practitioner and policymakers to adopt and implement the recommended changes.

Activities

REFLECTION

1. Spend 10 minutes reflecting on the benefits of becoming aware of the historical aspects of cultural competence.

CLINICAL ENCOUNTERS OF HUMANS AND NONHUMANS

- Take a moment to think about a clinical encounter you have had with a patient from a cultural background different than your own.

- Summarize the encounter in two to three sentences.
- In the center of your paper, write the word and draw a circle around it.
- Next, start mapping out the various human and nonhuman actors/forces that may have influenced this cross-cultural clinical encounter.
- Represent each one with a circle or shape radiating out from the center.
- Once you have identified key human and nonhuman elements, start drawing connections between them to illustrate relationships, tensions, negotiations, etc.
- Spend a few minutes studying your map and then reflect on:
  - Nonhuman forces you may have overlooked.
  - Elements that seem most influential or problematic.
  - Potential opportunities to redesign/renegotiate human–nonhuman relationships for more culturally competent care.

REFERENCES

Ang, S., & van Dyne, L. (Eds.). (2008). *Handbook of cultural intelligence. Theory, measurement and applications*. M.E Sharpe.

Aristotle. (2004). *Nicomachean ethics. Book II*. Penguin Classics.

Bennett, M. J. (1986). A developmental approach to training for intercultural sensitivity. *International Journal of Intercultural Relations, 10*(2), 179–196.

Berlin, E., & Fowkes, W. (1982). A teaching framework for cross-cultural health care. *Western Journal of Medicine, 139*(6), 934–938.

Cross, T., Bazron, B., Dennis, K., & Issacs, M. (1989). *Towards a culturally competent system of care: A monograph on effective services for minority children who are severely emotionally disturbed. Vol 1*. Georgetown University Child Development Centre.

Earley, C. P., & Ang, S. (2003). *Cultural intelligence: Individual interactions across cultures*. Stanford Business Books.

Ferrando, F. (2023). Existential posthumanism: A manifesto. In R. Braidotti, E. Jones, & G. Klumbytė (Eds.), *More posthuman glossary*. Bloomsbury.

Gelfand, J., Imai, L., & Fehr, R. (2008). Thinking intelligently about cultural intelligence: The road ahead. In S. Ang, & L. van Dyne (Eds.), *Handbook of cultural intelligence*. Theory, measurement and applications. M.E Sharpe.

Hall, E. T. (1959). *The silent language*. Anchor.

Hofstede, G. (1980). *Culture's consequences: International differences in work-related values*. SAGE Publications.

Kelley, T. L. (1927). *Interpretation of educational measurements*. World Book Company.

Leininger, M. (1995). Transcultural nursing perspectives. Basic concepts, principles, and culture care incidents. In M. Leininger, & M. R. McFarland (Eds.), *Transcultural nursing: Concepts, theories, research and practice* (2nd ed., pp. 57–92). McGraw Hill.

Office of Minority Health. (2013). *National standards for culturally and linguistically appropriate services in health and health care*. U.S. Department of Health and Human Services.

Papadopoulos, I., Taylor, G., Ali, S., Aagard, M., Akman, O., Alpers, L. M., Apostolara, P., Biglete-Pangilinan, S., Biles, J., García, Á. M., González-Gil, T., Koulouglioti, C., Kouta, C., Krepinska, R., Kumar, B. N., Lesińska-Sawicka, M., Diaz, A. L. L., Malliarou, M., Nagórska, M., & Zorba, A. (2017). Exploring nurses' meaning and experiences of compassion: An international online survey involving 15 countries. *Journal of Transcultural Nursing, 28*(3), 286–295.

Papadopoulos I. (2018). Culturally competent compassion: Aguide for healthcare students and practitioners. Routledge, London and New York.

Papadopoulos, I., Lazzarino, R., Koulouglioti, C., Aagard, M., Akman, Ö., Alpers, L. M., Apostolara, P., Araneda Bernal, J., Biglete-Pangilinan, S., Eldar-Regev, O., González-Gil, M. T., Kouta, C., Krepinska, R., Lesińska-Sawicka, M., Liskova, M., Lopez-Diaz, A. L., Malliarou, M., Martín-García, Á., Muñoz-Salinas, M., & Zorba, A. (2020). Obstacles to compassion-giving among nursing and midwifery managers: An international study. *International Nursing Review, 67*(4), 437–567.

Papadopoulos, I., Lazzarino, R., Koulouglioti, C., & Wright, S. (2022). Towards a national strategy for the provision of spiritual care during major health disasters: A qualitative study. *International Journal of Health Planning and Management, 37*(4), 1990–2006.

Papadopoulos, I., Tilki, M., & Taylor, G. (1998). *Transcultural care. A guide for health care professionals.* Quay Books.

Papadopoulos, I. (2006). *Transcultural health and social care: Development of culturally competent practitioners.* Churchill Livingstone Elsevier.

Spector, R. E. (2017). *Cultural diversity in health and illness* (9th ed.). Pearson.

Sue, D. W., & Sue, D. (2016). *Counselling the culturally diverse: Theory and practice* (7th ed.). John Wiley & Sons Inc.

Tervalon, M., & Murray-Garcia, J. (1998). Cultural humility versus cultural competence: A critical distinction in defining physician training outcomes in multicultural education. *Journal of Health Care for the Poor and Underserved, 9*(2), 117.

United Nations General Assembly. (1948). *Universal Declaration of Human Rights (UDHR).* United Nations General Assembly. https://www.un.org/en/universal-declaration-human-rights/.

Van Oudenhoven, J. P., & Van der Zee, K. I. (2002). Predicting multicultural effectiveness of international students: The multicultural personality questionnaire. *International Journal of Intercultural Relations, 26*(6), 679–694.

WHO. (2008). *Closing the gap in a generation: Health equity through action on the social determinants of health.* World Health Organisation.

WHO. (2019). *Monitoring health inequality: An essential step for achieving health equity.* World Health Organisation.

Chapter 3

Key Concepts: The Big Six Cs

Learning Objectives

After reading this chapter, you should be more informed about the following concepts and how they relate to culturally competent and compassionate nursing and allied health care:

- Communication
- Compassion
- Courage
- Collaboration.
- Cybernetics
- Connectivity

Introduction

The true essence of humanity lies in the profound dance of communication, where words intertwine with understanding, compassion guides hearts, courage fuels noble endeavours, collaboration weaves the fabric of progress, cybernetics unveils the harmony of man and machine, and connectivity binds us in the symphony of shared existence. (Anon)

This chapter expands on some of the key concepts that form the building blocks of cultural competence and compassion. The chapter begins with the recognition that despite the challenges that exist in our increasingly interconnected world, the ability to effectively communicate across cultural boundaries has become essential. It continues with a deep exploration of the meanings and importance of compassion, which is inextricably linked to cultural competence. Next comes the concept of courage, identified as a virtue that complements compassion. The significance of collaboration as the vehicle carrying and delivering the actions related to the previous key concepts will be explored from different angles using a similar approach as for the previous key concepts. A new topic that carries both virtues and principles is that of posthumanism. In this chapter, we will explore the notion of cybernetics and its relation to cultural competence. The chapter concludes by bringing together the key concepts in order to discuss the significance of the connectivity of humans, nonhuman entities, and the environment.

In this and almost all other chapters in this book, I am including relevant philosophical thoughts from the ancient and modern eras as well as theories from other disciplines. I believe that the historical context helps the reader appreciate the evolution of nursing thought and how it has been shaped by different philosophical traditions. On the other hand, interdisciplinary connections enrich nursing knowledge. They can illustrate how nursing concepts are interconnected with broader concepts and principles. This interdisciplinary approach fosters a more comprehensive understanding of nursing and encourages both students and qualified nurses to think critically about the diverse influences that shape nursing practice. I believe that by presenting multiple philosophical perspectives, both ancient and modern, as well as examples from other disciplines, it can inspire the readers to develop their own informed understanding of the essential concepts of nursing.

Communication

DEFINING COMMUNICATION

Intercultural and cross-cultural communication refers to the communication process between individuals or groups from different cultural backgrounds. It involves understanding and navigating the diverse perspectives, values, norms, and communication styles that exist across cultures.

ANCIENT AND MODERN PHILOSOPHERS' VIEWS ON COMMUNICATION

Ancient and modern philosophers have offered various perspectives on communication, highlighting its significance, challenges, and ethical dimensions. For example, the Greek philosopher Plato (428–348 BCE) emphasized the importance of clear and truthful communication (Plato, 1991). He also warned us of the potential for manipulation and deception and pointed the need for ethical communication rooted in truth and justice.

Another Greek philosopher, Aristotle (384–322 BCE), identified three key elements of persuasive communication: *ethos* (credibility), *pathos* (emotion), and *logos* (logic) (Aristotle, 1989). Aristotle believed that communication should aim to achieve a balance of these elements to effectively persuade and engage the audience.

The Chinese philosopher Confucius (551–479 BCE) emphasized the importance of ethical communication and interpersonal relationships (Confucius, 1979). He stressed the value of respectful dialogue, empathy, and listening to others. According to Confucius, effective communication is rooted in the virtue of benevolence and contributes to the harmonious functioning of society.

The ancient examples about communication were wise and timeless. The modern philosophers and scholars added their own views on the importance of communication. For example, the anthropologist Edward T. Hall (1914–2009) studied the ways in which culture influences communication. In his book 'Silent language' he argued that culture is a form of silent language that shapes how we interact and perceive the world (Hall, 1959). He also discussed the different ways cultures perceive and use time, space, and gestures/body language. Overall, Hall emphasized a deep understanding of cultural contexts, both one's own and others', in order to improve communication and avoid misunderstandings in an increasingly interconnected world. According to him, paying attention to unspoken cultural norms is key.

The German theologist Martin Buber's (1878–1965) philosophy centred around the concept of 'I–Thou' relationships, which can be between two individuals or between a tree, the sky, an animal, God, and other entities (Buber, 1970). Buber believed that genuine communication occurs when individuals acknowledge and engage with each other as unique and equal beings.

Mikhail Bakhtin's (1895–1975) dialogic theory of communication emphasized the social nature of language and communication (Bakhtin, 1981). He viewed communication as a dynamic and interactive process that creates meaning through the exchange of diverse voices and perspectives. Bakhtin emphasized the importance of open dialogue and the recognition of multiple viewpoints.

Jürgen Habermas (1929–) developed the concept of communicative action, highlighting the role of communication in the construction of social reality and democratic processes (Habermas, 1984, 1987). He argued that open, inclusive, and rational communication among individuals is essential for a just and democratic society.

Gayatri Chakravorty Spivak (1942–) is known for her work on postcolonial theory and deconstruction (Spivak, 2010). Spivak has written extensively about intercultural communication, arguing that it is important to recognize the power dynamics that exist between different cultures.

Naomi Scheman's (1946–) work focuses on feminist theory, pragmatism, and the philosophy of language (Scheman, 2011). She has written extensively about intercultural communication, arguing that it is important to be aware of the ways in which our own culture shapes our understanding of other cultures.

These philosophers offer diverse insights into the nature and significance of communication, highlighting its role in conveying knowledge, building relationships, shaping social realities, and promoting ethical and democratic interactions. Their perspectives continue to inform discussions on effective communication, rhetoric, interpersonal relationships, and the impact of communication technologies in contemporary society. All of them are relevant in culturally competent nursing, as well as healthcare in general.

POSTHUMAN THEORY AND COMMUNICATION

Haraway (2016) defines posthumanism as an ethical position that extends moral concern to things that are different from us, the humans, in particular to other species and objects with which we cohabit in this world. The interconnectedness between humans and nonhuman entities is evident in many ancient cultures. For example, Watts (2013) examined the North American indigenous worldviews that recognize nonhuman agencies, mandating respectful, ethical relations between all components of the living world. She goes on to express her concerns about how modern times and societies were corrupted, believing that humans are the superior beings on our planet, based on their intelligence and ability to communicate. However, the 21st century ushered in the era of deep thinking and critiquing of the superiority of humans over other species and the growing existence of nonhuman entities.

Let us now examine the contemporary views of the posthuman theorists about communication. Posthumanists argue that human language and communication should be understood as continuous with the signaling and information exchange found in other living beings and even technologies. Posthumanist scholars see communication as a complex, multimodal, embodied process that operates beyond human-centered frameworks. Communication emerges through dynamic connections between diverse human and nonhuman actors. Communication is viewed as an ethical relation for negotiating differences, deconstructing anthropocentric assumptions, and building meaningful possesses across species and systems. Posthumanism asks us to remember our true place in the world, which is to be an integral part of nature (Oberauer, 2021). Recognizing the interdependence of species highlights the importance of fostering harmonious relationships rather than asserting superiority.

Human language and speech are undoubtedly complex and sophisticated forms of communication, allowing for the expression of abstract thoughts, sharing of knowledge, and managing complex social interactions. However, it is important to recognize that animals also communicate through various means, such as vocalizations, body language, chemical signals, and even sophisticated systems of communication among certain species.

CHALLENGES AND BARRIERS IN INTERCULTURAL COMMUNICATION

Communication with patients of diverse cultural backgrounds is of utmost importance in healthcare settings. Effective communication in these situations ensures that patients receive the best possible care, improves patient satisfaction, fosters trust and rapport, and reduces the risk of misunderstandings and medical errors.

To achieve effective communication, health and care workers must be aware that cultures differ in their communication styles, ranging from direct to indirect, also described as linear and straightforward communication (direct), or storytelling and context dependent communication (indirect). For example, my cultural roots derive from my Greek Cypriot culture. My preferred communication style is that of storytelling, context dependent. When I am listening to people, especially those who come from a different cultural background to mine, I like to hear the context of the message they are transmitting; likewise, when I am talking to a person, irrespective of their cultural background, I use my natural storytelling style,

which helps me build rapport before conveying the key message. This invariably requires more time than using the direct linear style. Busy health and care workers have been professionally acculturated to believe that the linear style is more efficient timewise. This is not always the case, since lack of sufficient context can hamper the patient care and may even result in dangerous misunderstandings. Limited time for communication can lead to rushed interactions, incomplete information sharing, and patients feeling unheard or dismissed. Allocating sufficient time for effective communication is essential for building trust and addressing patient concerns.

Linked to the importance of cultural context is that of language differences, which can pose significant challenges and barriers in intercultural communication. Translating words alone is not sufficient; understanding cultural nuances and idiomatic expressions is essential for effective communication.

Another crucial element of communication is that of interpreting the nonverbal cues such as gestures, facial expressions, eye contact, tone of voice, and personal space, all of which may vary across cultures. To avoid their misinterpretation, the culturally competent health and care worker must respectfully and compassionately ask the patient to verify their understanding of the nonverbal signals or ask for an explanation.

A culturally competent caregiver, leader, educator, and manager understands that preconceived notions and stereotypes can hinder effective intercultural communication. Stereotyping can lead to biased judgments that can have a negative impact on the health and well-being of both patients and caregivers.

While getting a good grip on the many theories of communication is essential to health

BOX 3.1 THE TOP 10 TIPS FOR INTERCULTURAL COMMUNICATION

1. Be mindful of your assumptions, biases, and stereotypes.
2. Do not discriminate or stigmatize.
3. Be tolerant to other cultures but also be culturally aware.
4. Be respectful and mindful of cultural differences.
5. Do not ignore other people's cultures but show an interest in them.
6. Ask questions and seek clarification.
7. Be an active listener and mindful of body language.
8. Be ready to learn new things.
9. Avoid slang and dialects.
10. Be self-aware and open minded.

and care sector staff, some practical tips on how to deliver intercultural communication are of equal importance. A colleague and I asked a group of final-year nursing students to come up with their top 10 tips for effective intercultural communication. Box 3.1 lists these practical tips.

Let us now apply these 10 tips for intercultural communication.

CASE STUDY: CULTURAL COMPETENCE AND COMMUNICATION CHALLENGES

Mr. Lopez, a 65-year-old man from Colombia, has been admitted to the hospital for treatment of a chronic respiratory condition. He speaks limited English and is accompanied by his son, who acts as his primary translator. During his hospital stay, Mr. Lopez experienced difficulties in communicating his needs and concerns to the healthcare team. Despite the presence of his son as a translator, there were instances of miscommunication and misunderstandings.

In order to overcome these challenges, the aforementioned 10 tips can be applied as recommended as follows:

1. Be mindful of your assumptions, biases, and stereotypes: The nursing staff consciously avoid making assumptions about Mr. Lopez's cultural beliefs or preferences based on stereotypes. They recognize the diversity within cultural groups and approach each patient as an individual.
2. Do not discriminate or stigmatize: Nurses treat Mr. Lopez with respect and dignity, ensuring that he receives the same level of care and attention as any other patient, regardless of his cultural background or language barriers.
3. Be tolerant to other cultures but also be culturally aware: The nurses acknowledge and respect Mr. Lopez's cultural beliefs and practices while also educating themselves about potential cultural influences on his health behaviors and possible beliefs that may harm him.
4. Be respectful and mindful of cultural differences: When interacting with Mr. Lopez, the nurses speak slowly and clearly, using simple language and avoiding complex medical jargon. They may also use pictures and maintain appropriate eye contact and body language.
5. Do not ignore other people's cultures but show an interest in them: The nurses ask Mr. Lopez and his son about their cultural practices, beliefs, and preferences related to healthcare. They express genuine interest in learning and understanding his cultural background to provide appropriate care.
6. Ask questions and seek clarification: If there is any confusion or miscommunication, the nurses should not hesitate

to ask clarifying questions or request additional explanations from Mr. Lopez or his son or from a professional interpreter. They encourage open dialogue and ensure that everyone is on the same page.

7. Be an active listener and mindful of body language: The nurses actively listen to Mr. Lopez and his son, paying attention not only to their words but also to their body language and nonverbal cues. They make the effort to understand the underlying messages and emotions being conveyed.

8. Be ready to learn new things: The healthcare team approaches Mr. Lopez's case with an open mind, recognizing that they may encounter cultural beliefs or practices that are new to them. They are willing to learn and adapt their care strategies as needed.

9. Avoid slang and dialects: When communicating with Mr. Lopez and his son, the nurses use clear, standard language, avoiding slang or colloquial expressions that could lead to misunderstandings.

10. Be self-aware and open-minded: The nurses remain self-aware of their own cultural biases and preconceptions, actively working to set them aside and approach each interaction with an open and non-judgmental mindset.

Through their culturally competent practices, the nursing team aims to build a trusting relationship with Mr. Lopez and his family, facilitating effective communication and ensuring that his cultural needs are respected and addressed throughout his hospital stay.

Different styles of communication, different languages, nonverbal cues, stereotypes, use of technical jargon, and lack of time and other resources represent some of the many challenges and barriers to effective intercultural communication. Understanding these barriers is crucial. Even though healthcare staff are very resourceful and now have the help of the new artificial intelligence (AI) technologies, they remain in need of training on intercultural communication and cultural competence. This will enhance their skills and booster their confidence, which will result in an acceptable level of communication in the increasingly multicultural health and care settings.

Compassion

DEFINING COMPASSION

I have defined culturally competent compassion as a human quality of understanding the suffering of others and wanting to do something about it using culturally appropriate and acceptable caring interventions that take into consideration both the patients' and the carers' cultural backgrounds as well as the context in which care is given (Papadopoulos, 2011, 2018).

The term *compassion* means ''to suffer with', from the Latin *com* (together with) and *pati* (to suffer) (Schantz, 2007). It has been suggested that compassion has its origins in religious ideologies (Armstrong, 2011; Straughair, 2012), and it is also a central focus of many spiritual and ethical traditions, from Buddhism to Confucianism to Christianity (Goetz et al., 2010). However, as we will see in this chapter, compassion has been a characteristic of humans and animals for millennia. In fact, there is growing scientific evidence that suggests that the human brain may be innately wired for compassion. Researchers have identified parts of the brain that are activated during altruistic and empathetic behavior, providing clues into the neurobiological basis of our capacity for caring about the welfare of others.

SCIENTIFIC EVIDENCE ABOUT COMPASSION

One of the most well-known studies was conducted by Jordan Grafman and colleagues in 2006. They used functional magnetic resonance imaging (fMRI) to scan the brains of volunteers as they were asked to envision different charitable giving scenarios. The researchers found that envisioning making a charitable donation activated the meso-limbic pathway, a reward-related circuitry in the brain (Grafman & Krueger, 2009). This suggests that our brains may reinforce compassionate acts by releasing dopamine and creating a sense of satisfaction.

Multiple studies associate altruistic behaviors like donating and volunteering time with activation in the subgenual anterior cingulate cortex and septal area, regions linked to social bonding, emotional regulation, and affiliation (Harbaugh et al., 2007; Moll et al., 2006). This suggests that acts of compassion may strengthen neural pathways for social connection, reinforcing our human instinct for cooperation.

The accumulating research on the neuroscience of compassion indicates that the brain may have evolved specific circuits to support altruistic behaviors such as compassion. While environmental and social factors play a key role, our capacity for compassion appears to have roots in our basic brain wiring (Grafman et al., 2009; Morelli et al., 2017; Rizzolatti & Fabbri-Destro, 2010).

BRIEF PHILOSOPHICAL EXPLANATIONS OF COMPASSION IN ANCIENT TIMES

Confucius (551–479 BC), the Chinese teacher, politician, and philosopher, declared that wisdom, compassion, and courage are the three universally recognized qualities of humans, emphasizing that people should have compassion toward each other (Confucius, 1979). In order to be compassionate, people should avoid self-aggrandizement and practice altruism and self-restraint (http://confucius-1.com/teachings/). His philosophy emphasized personal morality, justice, sincerity, and correct social relationships. Confucius taught that the heart–mind defines the uniqueness of being human, and thus he insisted on empathizing and extending virtues to others as a method of cultivating humanity.

Confucius' social philosophy was based on 'ren', a concept akin to the notions of loving, kindness, benevolence, goodness, and humaneness. His golden rule was: "*Do not do to others what you would not like them do to you*" (Low, 2011). *Ren* is concerned with the belief that the greatest value in life is selfless dedication to one's community.

Confucius' political beliefs were further based on the concept of self-discipline. He believed that a leader needed to demonstrate self-discipline and provide a positive example in order to remain humble and treat his followers with compassion (Box 3.2).

The Greek philosopher Aristotle (384–322 BC) gives pride of place to compassion as an emotional virtue, describing it as the experience of pain of another person's undeserved bad fortune (Kristjánsson, 2014; Aristotle, 2004). Aristotle conceived the individual's reaction to tragedy as a combination of fear and compassion directed toward the pain of another being. Thus, for there to be compassion, we need to acknowledge a situation as something harmful for the other, recognizing at the same time that although this person is

BOX 3.2 KEY POINTS OF CONFUCIUS' PHILOSOPHY ON COMPASSION

- Confucius focused on how individuals should live their lives and interact with others.
- He placed much emphasis on benevolence as the most important characteristic of human beings.
- Confucius' philosophy was based on 'ren' (loving others), and he was the founder of the golden rule (Do not do to others what you would not like them do to you).
- He believed that a good leader needed to exercise self-discipline in order to treat his followers with compassion.
- The guiding principle in Confucius' social teachings is that people should love one another and treat each other with kindness.

BOX 3.3 KEY POINTS OF ARISTOTLE'S PHILOSOPHY ON COMPASSION

- Aristotle describes compassion as an emotional virtue, defining it as pain at another person's undeserved bad fortune.
- Aristotle conceived the individual's reaction to tragedy as a combination of fear and compassion directed toward the pain of another being.
- He recognized that what befalls one person could befall any of us.
- Aristotle perceived compassion as being worthy to those who are undeserving of suffering.

different from us, our shared humanity and vulnerability become a common bond.

Saunders (2015) argues that Aristotle's use of the word 'pity' is clearly a reference to compassion as outlined in the Aristotelian definition of pity as a feeling of pain at an apparent evil, which is destructive or painful, that befalls one who does not deserve it and which we might expect to befall ourselves or some friend of ours.

Aristotle prioritized appraisals of deservingness, rooted in assumptions regarding the sufferer's character and intentions. He defined compassion as an emotion directed at others' suffering and indicated three necessary factors: perceiving others' suffering seriously, believing this suffering is not deserved, and believing that any one of us could suffer from the same event (Taner, n.d.) (Box 3.3).

BRIEF PHILOSOPHICAL EXPLANATIONS OF COMPASSION IN MODERN TIMES

The American philosopher Martha Nussbaum (2001) argues in her book *Upheavals of Thought: The Intelligence of Emotions* that compassion is an important moral emotion that involves recognizing the suffering of others, seeing their condition as serious, and believing it could happen to oneself or one's own loved ones. She states that cultivating compassion creates a bridge of concern between people. Nussbaum's definition is very similar to that provided by Aristotle.

A different kind of compassion worth a brief description is that of Kristin Neff (2023), a scholar who coined the term 'self-compassion'. She identified three key components of it:

- Self-kindness: Being kind, understanding, and forgiving toward oneself, rather than harshly judgmental. Not berating oneself for imperfections.
- Common humanity: Viewing one's experiences as part of the shared human condition rather than isolating. Recognizing all people have struggles.
- Mindfulness: Holding one's painful thoughts and emotions with balanced awareness rather than overidentifying with them.

Neff views self-compassion as distinct from self-esteem. Self-compassion is warmer, more connected to others, and more forgiving than simply esteeming oneself positively.

She proposes self-compassion can be developed through practices like loving-kindness meditation, keeping self-compassion journals, and actively soothing oneself in difficult times through touch, words, etc. Having compassion for oneself allows for recognizing destructive behaviors without condemning one's core self-worth.

In summary, Neff sees self-compassion as the antidote to harmful self-judgment and a key pathway to inner peace. Her research validates self-compassion as a powerful therapeutic tool (Neff et al., n.d.).

EVIDENCE FROM A RESEARCH STUDY

In 2014, stimulated by the public and scholarly debates in the United Kingdom about care without compassion, I decided to undertake an investigation into some of the issues around this topic that both the public and the professionals appeared to agree upon.

I wanted to establish whether or not this topic interested nurses globally and whether or not there were cultural similarities and differences with the issues that had emerged in the United Kingdom. To start with, I created a 10-question survey questionnaire that was piloted by 73 South Korean nurses. The survey was administered online in the languages of the partner countries. A total of 1323 nurses from 15 countries completed the compassion survey (Papadopoulos et al., 2017).

The survey generated a large set of quantitative and qualitative data. Each country's responses to the open-ended questions were sent to the respective coresearchers for translation and quality checks of accuracy and meaning. All translated data were sent to the UK team for in-depth country and comparative analysis.

THE RESULTS

The majority of participants defined compassion as a deep awareness of the suffering of others and a wish to alleviate it. Other definitions worth reporting here were as follows:

- Being able to see the others as equal and include them with respect in their sadness, in their joy, in their adversity, or in their walk through life, never from a moralistic perspective but with an attitude of solidarity (Colombian participant)
- Good and equal care (Turkish Cypriot participant)
- Empathy in the spirit of following the emotions of the other person, effort to connect to the person, and effort to find together a path to mitigate the problems of his or her suffering (Czech Republic participant)

The analysis revealed that participants considered compassion as a conscious and intentional act consisting of a list of components and actions. These are shown in Figure 3.1. The components were as follows:

A. <u>Time:</u> Nurses reported making conscious efforts to overcome the constraints of time. An Australian participant stated that making patients feel that their suffering is worthy of the nurses' time is very important, while a Greek nurse expressed the view that compassion is about devoting time to be with the patients and simply hold their hand when they are in pain.

B. <u>Being there:</u> An American nurse explained that recognizing the important times for the patients and being there for them is crucial and comforting. A nurse from the Czech Republic described a similar sentiment stating that nurses should be able to express compassion in the moment.

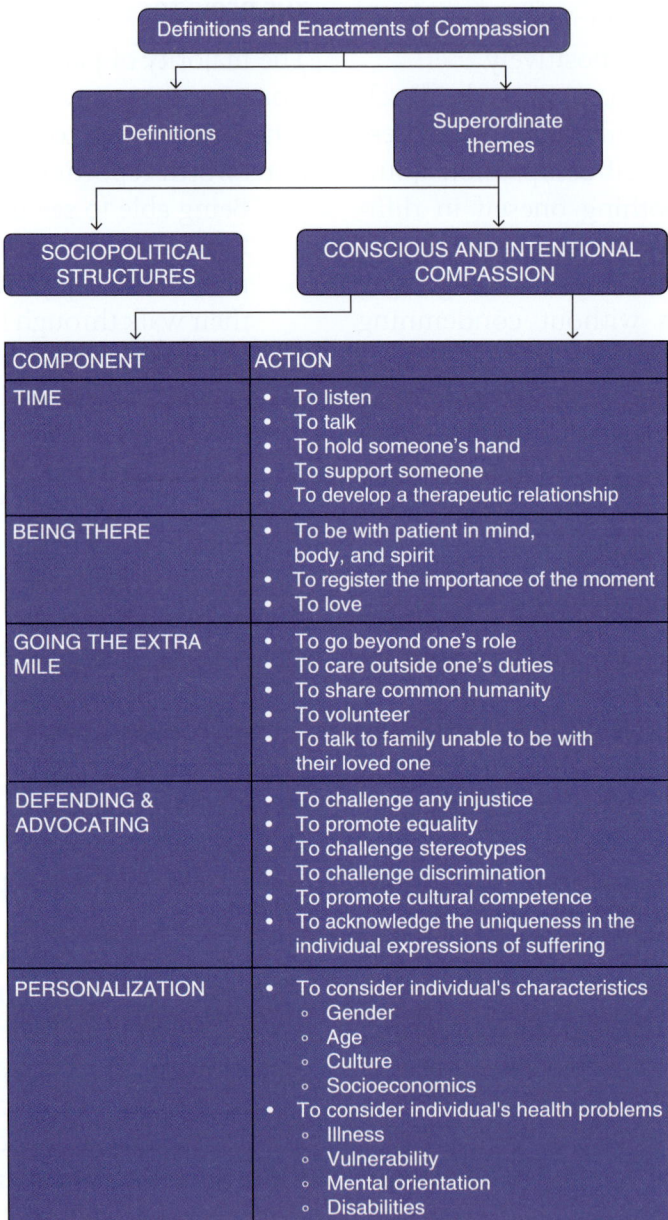

Figure 3.1 Culturally competent compassion—components and actions.

C. <u>Going the extra mile:</u> Giving extra time to a lonely patient, doing acts of benevolence that go beyond one's job, making a phone call to ask about the transition from hospital to home were examples given by Italian, Norwegian, Spanish, and Colombians participants, some of whom also suggested that maybe some of these acts by nurses are done not because they are part of their job but because they are compassionate human beings.

D. Defending and advocating: Many participants stated that protecting the human rights of vulnerable people was central to compassionate practice. A participant from Turkey suggested that nurses listen to patients and their families actively trying to understand their problems, pain, anger, or love, in order to defend them.

E. Personalization: A participant from Israel wrote that nurses should understand that each person's suffering is subjective and unique, while a participant from Philippines stated that compassion requires cultural awareness.

LEARNING TO BE A COMPASSIONATE NURSE

The majority of the participant (97%) declared that compassion is important in nursing. Nearly 60% believed that compassion can be taught to nurses, while a quarter of the participants (25%) did not believe that it can. However, while only 11% of the participants reported that the correct amount of compassion content was being taught, many more (44%) reported that not enough was being taught. In terms of important influences in developing compassion, the participants were almost equally divided between these three influences: the family, the individual cultural values, and the personal experiences of compassion.

RECEIVING COMPASSION AT WORK

Almost 50% of the participants reported that that they receive compassion from patients. A further 46% reported to be receiving compassion from colleagues. Sadly, only 4% reported receiving compassion from their managers. This significant finding was reported by all participants, with the exception of those from Philippines and the Turkish-speaking Cypriots.

In conclusion, the findings suggest that one's country of residence, cultural background, personal experiences, and the context of their work influence the way they define compassion. The findings clearly indicate the need for inclusion of culturally competent compassion within the education programs of nurses.

A more extensive reporting of the qualitative and quantitative data from this study can be found in two published articles (Papadopoulos et al., 2016, 2017).

Courage

DEFINING COURAGE

Courage has been defined as the wilful choice to pursue virtuous actions despite risks to one's self-interest (Pianalto, 2012). It involves acting on one's ethical beliefs when the personally expedient path would be to remain silent or disengaged. Scholars have delineated different facets of courage relevant to cultural competence in healthcare. For example:

Moral courage: Speaking up for what is right despite fear of adverse consequences (Kidder, 2009; Murray, 2010).

Psychological courage: Facing our deep-seated fear of psychological instability (Putman, 1997).

Intellectual courage: Challenging existing knowledge paradigms and integrating new, complex ideas (Pianalto, 2012).

Civil courage: Publicly supporting just causes through collective action (Greitemeyer et al., 2006).

All these forms of courage should be part of the skills each healthcare professional and healthcare-providing institutions must develop and practice, especially those who aspire to be culturally competent or wish to enhance their level of cultural competence.

THE EVOLUTION OF THE MEANING OF COURAGE

Courage has been extensively explored by philosophers across cultures and eras. While universal in essence, perspectives on courage have evolved over time, as thinkers have aimed to define its qualities and relation to human flourishing.

ANCIENT PERSPECTIVES ON COURAGE

In ancient Greece, courage was deemed one of the four cardinal virtues, along with wisdom, temperance, and justice.

Plato (427–347 BCE) believed that true courage is not merely the absence of fear but also the ability to control and overcome one's irrational desires, guided by reason and virtue (Plato, 1991).

Aristotle (384–322 BCE) described courage as a virtue that lies between recklessness and cowardice (Aristotle, 2004). He believed that courageous individuals strike a balance between being rash and being afraid, facing challenging situations with the right amount of confidence and fear.

Epicurus (341–270 BCE) viewed courage as the ability to overcome irrational fears and anxieties (Epicurus, 1993). For Epicurus, courage involved freeing oneself from unnecessary desires and fears, which he believed would lead to a state of ataraxia (tranquillity) and eudaimonia (happiness).

Each of these ancient Greek philosophers is highlighting in his unique perspectives the importance of self-control, balance, and mental resilience in facing life's challenges. Their contributions to the study of courage continues to influence philosophical discussions on ethics and human virtues.

TWENTIETH-CENTURY VIEWS ON COURAGE

The Indian politician and philosopher Mahatma Gandhi (1869–1948) was a man of great courage. He was willing to stand up for what he believed in, even when it was difficult or dangerous to do so. He used nonviolence as a tool to fight for justice and equality, and he inspired millions of people around the world with his example.

Here are some examples of Gandhi's courage (Gandhi, 1913):

He led the Salt March in 1930, a nonviolent protest against the British salt monopoly. He was arrested and imprisoned for his actions, but the protest was ultimately successful in drawing attention to the Indian independence movement.

Gandhi is credited with a number of quotes on courage, such as *"Courage is the virtue that guarantees all others."*

He was assassinated in 1948 by a Hindu extremist who disagreed with his views on religious tolerance. Gandhi never wavered in his commitment to nonviolence, even in the face of death.

Gandhi's legacy continues to inspire people today, and he remains one of the most important figures in the history of nonviolent resistance.

Martin Luther King, Jr. (1929–1968) was another man of great courage. Just like Gandhi, he was willing to stand up for what he believed in, even when it was difficult or dangerous to do so. He also used nonviolent resistance to fight for civil rights of African Americans, and he inspired millions of people around the world with his example.

In 1955, he became involved in the Montgomery bus boycott, a nonviolent protest against segregation on public buses. The boycott lasted for over a year and resulted in the desegregation of the Montgomery bus system. He went on to lead many other protests against segregation, including the March on Washington in 1963. In his famous "I Have a Dream" speech, he delivered a powerful message of hope and equality for all people. He continued to fight for civil rights until his assassination in 1968.

Here are some quotes from Martin Luther King, Jr. about courage:

Courage is not the absence of fear, but the triumph over it. The brave man is not he who does not feel afraid, but he who conquers that fear.

Injustice anywhere is a threat to justice everywhere.

Nelson Mandela (1918–2013) is considered to be the embodiment of courage and social justice. He dedicated his life to fighting against apartheid, the system of racial segregation in South Africa. He was imprisoned for 27 years for his beliefs, but he never gave up hope. He emerged from prison to lead the fight for a free and democratic South Africa, and he became the country's first Black president.

Mandela's courage was evident in many ways. He was willing to stand up to the apartheid government, even when it meant risking his life. He was also willing to forgive his enemies, and he worked to build a just and equitable society for all South Africans. (Mandela, 1994)

In his book *Long Walk to Freedom* (1994), Mandela wrote:

Time and again, I have seen men and women risk and give their lives for an idea. I have seen men stand up to attacks and torture without breaking, showing a strength and resilience that defies the imagination. I learned that courage was not the absence of fear, but the triumph over it. (p. 748)

One of the contemporary thinkers, philosopher, and professor of ethics and law, who has written extensively on courage, is the American Martha Nussbaum. She argues that courage is not simply about facing physical danger but also about facing moral challenges. She writes, "*Courage is not just about standing up to physical threats, but also about standing up to the threats of humiliation, degradation, and loss of self-respect*" (Nussbaum, 2001, p. 10).

Another contemporary thinker who has written about courage is Charles Taylor. In his book *The Ethics of Authenticity*, Taylor argues that courage is essential for living an authentic life. He writes, "*Courage is the capacity to stand up for what we believe in, even when it is difficult or dangerous to do so*" (Taylor, 1991, p. 77).

Other thinkers of our era have aimed to broaden and democratize courage (Pury et al., 2023). Murdoch (1993) portrays courage as the willingness to perceive others clearly with love and justice. Engster (2007) advocates democratic courage to uphold civic virtues and rights. Across eras, contemplating courage remains relevant for elucidating the human strengths needed to counter fear and live well together.

In my work on cultural competence and compassion, I emphasize the importance of courage in nursing practices. Here, I provide two examples.

The first example is that of providing compassion to patients, to their significant others, and to colleagues. In my view, nurses and other healthcare professional are often involved in sensitive, life-changing, and devastating situations that provoke in them fear, sadness, anxiety, and even panic. How can they tell a parent that their beloved child is dead or dying? How can they tell a young woman that she has an incurable type of cancer? How can they answer the questions of a chronically ill man who wishes to end his life and his suffering? Of course, the nurse or the doctor cannot walk away, but they must muster enough courage to manage their feelings and provide the necessary compassionate care. Reflecting on the exceptional as well as the everyday examples described earlier may inspire them to use a balanced amount of courage to deal with extreme situations in a sensitive, compassionate, and culturally appropriate way, without harming themselves.

My second example of nursing practice that requires courage is that of challenging prejudice, discrimination inequalities, oppression, racism, etc. All these forms of oppression and marginalization exist in the health and care sections and will continue to exist for various reasons. Nurses and other health professionals must not stay silent and passive when they witness discrimination or oppressive behaviors, rules, organizational plans, practices, and so on, whether these are direct or indirect overt or hidden. A culturally competent nurse must challenge these and must champion, through advocacy and speaking up, the eradication of all forms of discrimination for the benefit of patients, families, and colleagues. Deciding to do the right thing for the right reasons requires a lot of courage. We know from the literature that negative consequences have occurred and continue to occur to those who dare to be brave, just as it happened to the courageous individuals we read about in the earlier sections. But equally positive change also happens that benefits everyone, when the courageous person approaches these challenges with wisdom, balanced emotions, and measured arguments.

Collaboration

DEFINING COLLABORATION

In healthcare, collaboration involves coordination between healthcare professionals across disciplines and specialties to deliver comprehensive, integrated patient care. It includes interprofessional teams, information sharing between providers, and partnering with patients and families. Collaboration aims to provide coordinated care, centered around the patient for better outcomes, reduced errors, and improved efficiency and satisfaction.

In general, all successful collaborations, irrespective of their fields of work and the level of collaboration (local, national, global, and two people, group(s), public and private large institutions, global conglomerates), depend on cultural competence to guide a number of elements:

- Communication
- Mutual trust
- Technologies
- Complementary strengths and capabilities
- Participatory decision-making
- Cooperation
- Shared values
- Connectivity
- Cultural competence

Developing cultural competence requires collaboration among healthcare professionals, patients, families, and communities. Collaboration fosters information sharing, relationship building, and collective actions needed to provide equitable, patient-centered care across cultures.

COLLABORATION IN ANCIENT TIMES

Collaboration has been the key to advancing knowledge, building civilizations, driving innovation, and tackling large-scale projects throughout human history. Philosophers and thinkers have extensively collaborated as well.

In ancient Egypt, collaboration is seen in the massive projects of the ancient Egyptians like the pyramids, which required thousands of laborers, architects, engineers, and priests to work together. The ancient Greek philosophers like Socrates, Plato, and Aristotle used a different type of collaboration that entailed building upon each other's ideas in the development of Western philosophy and science. In Baghdad and Muslim Spain around 900–1200 CE, Islamic scholars collaborated significantly to advance medicine, mathematics, and astronomy. On the remote Pacific islands, native Polynesians used highly advanced collaborative skills in navigating oceans, combining astronomy, marine biology, and geography to undertake voyages (Finney, 1976; Guthrie, 1950; Lyons, 2010; Mark, 2017).

COLLABORATION IN MODERN TIMES

There are plenty of examples of collaborations in modern times that clearly show how much humans can achieve if they connect and collaborate. Of course, we must not forget or undermine the daily collaborations between individuals and groups who also contribute to humanity, but here I would like to list collaborations that have changed our modern world.

- The Human Genome Project was an international research collaboration to sequence and map the human genome, which enabled discoveries in diseases, medical interventions, as well as therapies for prevention of diseases and many more benefits. This longitudinal study involved scientists from 20+ countries (Collins, 2003).
- Scientists from across the world collaborate on the largest particle physics laboratory at the European Council for Nuclear Research (CERN) to study fundamentals of physics. CERN Large Hadron Collider is a collaboration of over 10,000 scientists and engineers from over 100 countries that contributed to building the particle collider and conducting experiments using it (Heuer, 2023; Overbye, 2022).
- The International Space Station (ISS) https://en.wikipedia.org/wiki/International_Space_Station is a collaboration between the space agencies of the United States, Russia, Canada, Europe, and Japan that built and operate the space station. Over 200 astronauts from 19 countries have worked aboard the ISS (ISS, n.d.).
- United Nations: An intergovernmental organization founded in 1945 as a global collaborative forum to promote peace, security, and international cooperation. It has 193 member states (United Nations, n.d.).
- Wikipedia: The online encyclopedia, cofounded by Jimmy Wales and Larry Sanger, was established in January

2001. Wikipedia is a free online platform. It allows users to create and edit articles collaboratively. Since its genesis, Wikipedia has grown into one of the largest and most widely used reference sources on the Internet, with articles on a wide range of topics contributed by volunteers from around the world. Anyone can edit and contribute to articles (https://en.wikipedia.org/wiki/History_of_Wikipedia).

- GAVI, the Vaccine Alliance: Created in 2000, GAVI is an international organization—a global vaccine alliance, bringing together public and private sectors with the shared goal of saving lives and protecting people's health by increasing equitable and sustainable use of vaccines. Access to immunization in poor countries is achieved through collaboration between organizations like the WHO, UNICEF, World Bank, vaccine companies, research institutes, and nongovernmental organizations (NGOs). GAVI collaborates with vaccine manufacturers to ensure the availability of affordable vaccines in low-income countries (https://www.gavi.org/our-alliance).

COLLABORATION IN HEALTH AND CARE SECTIONS

Collaboration in health and care involves healthcare providers, patients, families, and communities working together toward shared goals, shared knowledge, and shared meaning (Pecukonis et al., 2008). It goes beyond basic cooperation to entail shared power, responsibilities, and accountability between partners (D'Amour et al., 2005). Key aspects of collaboration for cultural competence include bidirectional communication in order to share

experiences and perspectives to build mutual understanding (Pecukonis et al., 2008), power sharing, and equal participation in decision-making and goal-setting (D'Amour et al., 2005), synergy, and reflexivity.

According to Banks and McGee Banks (2019), collaboration is an integral part of cultural competence with regard to understanding each partner's cultural backgrounds, values, practices, and needs. They also recommend that through collaboration diverse stakeholders can provide input to create culturally sensitive programs, processes, and facilities. Alizadeh and Chavan (2016) refer to the important collaboration between healthcare workers, patients, and families who can input valuable cultural information during all stages of treatment. Finally, D'Amour et al. (2005) explain that collaboration fosters trust and social capital that improve community health outcomes.

The benefits of collaboration are many, and therefore it is vital that nurses and other health-care workers are encouraged to work within multidisciplinary and multicultural collaborations such as research projects, patient panels, training courses, and so on, as this will enhance the quality of patient care (Box 3.4).

Cybernetics

Cybernetics is the study of control and communication in living beings and machines. It encompasses a wide range of interdisciplinary approaches, examining the flow of information within systems, the principles of self-regulation, and the interconnection of feedback loops between various components (Heims, 1991). Cybernetics emerged in the 1940s through the work of scientists like Norbert Wiener (1894–1964), who studied self-regulating systems. The term *cybernetics*

BOX 3.4 KEY POINTS ABOUT THE BENEFITS OF COLLABORATION

- Collaboration allows healthcare professionals, patients, families, and communities to pool their complementary expertise and insights to cocreate culturally competent and compassionate systems of care and build mutual understanding.
- Making collaboration a priority will also help develop a healthcare workforce ready to partner with diverse populations and address inequities.
- Overall, collaboration provides a critical foundation for lifelong growth in delivering culturally competent care (Alizadeh & Chavan, 2016; Brashers et al., 2020; D'Amour et al., 2005).

derives from the Greek word *kybernetis*, meaning "governor" or " ruler".

Key aspects of cybernetics include (Capra & Luisi, 2014) the following:

Circularity: Systems are circular and operate through feedback loops rather than linear cause–effect.

Holism: The whole system must be analyzed rather than just its constituent parts.

Adaptability: Systems self-organize and adapt to changing conditions.

A cyborg, short for "cybernetic organism", is a being that combines human parts, for example, a human liver, brain, heart, etc., as well as biomechatronic body parts, such as a robotic limb. The term is most commonly used to describe an organism that has enhanced abilities due to technology integrated with its body. The integration of an organism with human and nonhuman parts challenges the notions of identity and humanity, as well as creating a huge number of ethical dilemmas.

For many years, cyborgs were only fictional beings, but human curiosity and imagination propelled them from the book to our TV and cinema screens. Many of them became famous or infamous heroes/villains such as the Cybermen from *Doctor Who*, the Borg from *Star Trek*, and the Robocop. In the real world, cyborg technologies like prosthetic limbs, exoskeletons, and biosensors are slowly emerging, although the full realization of cyborgs with seamless integration between biological and digital systems requires more time and further research.

RELEVANCE OF CYBERNETICS TO CULTURAL COMPETENCE

Interestingly, the theory of cybernetics was developing at the same time as that of transcultural nursing and its later companion that of cultural competence. It is reasonable to suggest that transcultural nursing and cultural competence can inform the development of cybernetics, and vice versa.

For example, the cybernetics notion of contextual adaptation can provide ideas about how cultural competence can adapt to serve diverse patients and communities with distinct needs, values, and environments. Another example is about the cybernetic explanations on how systems and professional cultures extend norms through circular reinforcement (Kirmayer, 2012).

Currently, a number of biomechatronic devices are being implanted on humans. For example, cochlear implants are used to treat severe hearing loss or deafness. The cochlear implants are implanted in the inner ear to stimulate the auditory nerve and provide a sense of sound. Retinal implants are designed to restore vision in people with certain types of blindness.

They are implanted in the retina and stimulate the remaining functional cells to create visual perceptions. Pacemakers and implantable cardioverter defibrillators (ICDs) are implanted in the heart to regulate heart rhythm and deliver electrical shocks to correct life-threatening arrhythmias. Deep brain stimulation (DBS) devices are implanted in the brain to alleviate symptoms of movement disorders such as Parkinson's disease. Spinal cord stimulators (SCSs) are used to manage chronic pain by being implanted near the spinal cord to deliver electrical pulses that interfere with pain signals. Neuroprosthetic devices interface directly with the nervous system to restore function of individuals with spinal cord injuries or other neurological conditions. Bionic limbs with advanced technology and sensors can be controlled by the user's neural signals, providing a more natural and intuitive movement. Artificial pancreas is used to monitor blood glucose levels and to deliver insulin in people with diabetes. Neural implants for brain–computer interfaces (BCIs) enable direct communication between the brain and external devices, potentially allowing paralyzed individuals to control computers or robotic limbs through their thoughts.

Cybernetic technologies are increasing at a fast rate, and a larger range of them will inevitably become available for human enhancement. It is for this reason that culturally competent nurses and other health professionals must increase their knowledge and skills in cybernetics. As mentioned earlier, the benefits of this technology are plenty, but so are the ethical and cultural questions that require to be answered. Caring for patients who may benefit from cybernetic devices will require an assessment of their cultural values and beliefs in order to reach mutual understanding in regard to their acceptance as well as their reasons for their rejection.

Another challenge for culturally competent nursing and cybernetics is the possible creation of health inequalities. Cybernetic devices and their implantation in the human body are costly. In countries without a free national healthcare system, the cost of such technologies may be prohibitive, resulting in more suffering and even death in comparison to those living in countries which provide the devices free. Culturally competent and compassionate nursing adopts the principle of health equality based on the spirit of the common consensus—that health is a human right.

This section of the chapter has provided a simple overview of some of the key notions about cybernetics and how these can contribute to revolutionary enhancements of culturally competent and compassionate nursing and healthcare. Incorporating cybernetic perspectives into health profession education can equip providers with a broader lens for accelerating systemic change. Ultimately, the cybernetic worldview reinforces that cultural competence requires ongoing collaborative learning and continuous adaptation (Box 3.5).

Connectivity

DEFINING CONNECTIVITY

Connectivity is crucial for understanding the structure, function, and dynamics of complex systems in various scientific fields. In generic scientific terms, connectivity refers to the degree to which different components or

BOX 3.5 THE RELEVANCE OF CYBERNETICS TO CULTURAL COMPETENCE

- Cybernetics is the study of control and communication in living beings and machines.
- It encompasses a wide range of interdisciplinary approaches, examining the flow of information within systems, the principles of self-regulation, and the interconnection of feedback loops between various components (Heims, 1991).
- Cybernetics emerged in the 1940s through the work of scientists like Norbert Wiener (1894–1964), who studied self-regulating systems.
- The term "cybernetics" derives from the Greek word *kybernetis*, meaning "governor" or "ruler".
- A cyborg, short for "cybernetic organism", is a being that combines human parts, for example, a human liver, brain, heart, etc., as well as biomechatronic body parts such as a robotic limb.
- The theory of cybernetics was developing almost at the same time as that of transcultural nursing and its later companion that of cultural competence.
- It is reasonable to suggest that transcultural nursing and cultural competence can inform the development of cybernetics, and vice versa.
- Cybernetic technologies are increasing at a fast rate and a larger range of them will inevitably become available for human enhancement.
- It is for this reason that culturally competent nurses and other health professionals must increase their knowledge and skills in cybernetics.

involves studying social networks, communication patterns, and the flow of information in societies.

In computer science, connectivity is about the ability of devices, computers, or different systems to communicate and exchange data with each other through networks or protocols.

Ecological connectivity refers to the extent to which habitats and populations of organisms are connected or linked within a landscape. Connectivity is crucial for the movement of species, the exchange of genetic material, and the overall biodiversity and resilience of ecosystems.

ANCIENT CIVILIZATIONS AND CONNECTIVITY

Ancient civilizations did have notions related to connections, relationships, and interactions that could be loosely related to the idea of connectivity. Ancient cultures had their own ways of understanding interconnectedness, but the terminology and context were different from our contemporary usage of connectivity. For example, the ancient Greeks and Romans built extensive road networks that connected their cities and empires. These roads allowed for the movement of goods and people, which helped spread ideas and culture throughout the Mediterranean world.

The ancient Egyptians also built a sophisticated system of canals that connected the Nile River with the Red Sea. The ancient Chinese build the Silk Road. Traders were able to travel from one place to another, bringing with them new ideas and goods. This helped connect different cultures and create a more interconnected world.

elements within a system are interconnected, linked, or able to exchange information or resources.

In different fields, connectivity may have specific definitions and applications. For example, in social sciences, connectivity can refer to the degree of connectedness between individuals, social groups, or institutions. It

The ancient indigenous people believed that all things are interconnected and that we are all responsible for taking care of the earth and each other. This belief is reflected in their art, stories, and ceremonies, which help remind us of our place in the web of life. Aboriginal art in Australia often features images of animals, plants, and the land, all of which are seen as being interconnected.

Indigenous stories often tell of the journeys of heroes and heroines who traveled to different parts of the world, meeting new people and learning new things. These stories reflect the belief that all people are connected, regardless of their race, culture, or language.

Indigenous ceremonies often involve the use of music, dance, and storytelling to create a sense of connection between the participants and the natural world. For example, the First Nations people of Canada have a ceremony called the Round Dance, which is a way of celebrating the interconnectedness of all things.

CONNECTIVITY IN THE 21ST CENTURY

The concept of connectivity is still important today, but it has taken on a new meaning in the modern world. In the 21st century, connectivity is not just about the flow of goods and people. It is also about the flow of information and ideas, in ways that are different from those that were conducted in the past.

Anthropologists explain connectivity in human societies and cultures by studying the social networks of kinship ties, friendships, and how these bonds connect individuals into wider communities and collectives. They also study how the exchange of goods, ideas, and practices across geographic and cultural boundaries creates interconnections between societies.

Psychologists such as Baumeister and Leary (1995) proposed the belongingness hypothesis that humans have a fundamental motivation to form lasting positive connections and relationships. They argued that the need to belong is innate and drives much of human behaviour. In her article, "Positive Psychology: Social Connectivity and Its Role Within Mental Health Nursing," Macfarlane (2020) discusses the work of Pavey et al. (2011), who proposed that social connection is a concept relating to belonging and feeling close to others. In her view, this is a core psychological need that is necessary for life satisfaction. Our ability to effectively communicate through voice and nonverbal signs such as touch and facial expression enables us to connect with and care for each other.

MODERN TECHNOLOGY AND CONNECTIVITY

In the 21st century, we have unimaginably powerful technologies, among them the Internet, which has made possible for people all over the world to connect with each other in real time. This has created a global community where people can share ideas, learn from each other, and build relationships. Other benefits of connectivity in modern times are the breakdown of many barriers, the building of digital bridges, and the creation of a more just and equitable societies.

However, the recently published report, from the United Nations specialist agency ITU (International Telecommunication Union), *Global Connectivity Report 2022. Achieving universal and meaningful connectivity in the decade of action* (ITU, 2022), informs us that in the last 30 years, the number of Internet users surged from a few million to almost 5 billion. Yet, the potential remains untapped because one-third of humanity remains offline and many users enjoy only basic connectivity. Universal connectivity remains a distant prospect. Internet penetration has reached 95% of the population in only 13 countries. During the COVID-19 pandemic, lockdowns resulted in an immediate spike in Internet usage of around 30%. The pandemic demonstrated the need for humans to connect during such major disasters.

POSTHUMAN THEORIES AND CONNECTIVITY

In recent years, scholars across diverse fields are also increasingly recognizing the complex interdependencies among humans, nonhuman entities, and the broader environment.

The postmodern perspective of posthumanism contends—as mentioned in some of the chapters in this book—that humans, technology, and nature intersect rather than existing as separate categories (Haraway, 2016). Pickering (2010) provides a contemporary explanation of connectivity among humans, nonhumans, and nature in his *The Cybernetic Brain: Sketches of Another Future*.

Cybernetics view organisms and systems as circles of complex feedback loops, interconnected through flows of information (Pickering, 2010). Mitchell's (2009) complexity theory explains the nonlinear dynamics in complex adaptive systems like ecosystems, which cannot be reduced to simple causes and components. The philosopher Braidotti (2013) argues for a posthuman ethics based on recognizing continuities and kinships between humans, animals, machines, and the environment. As mentioned earlier in this chapter, the indigenous cultures around the world often have unique perspectives on the interconnectedness between humans and nature. The book *Braiding Sweetgrass: Indigenous Wisdom, Scientific Knowledge, and the Teachings of Plants* by Kimmerer (2013) provides insights into how indigenous peoples perceive their relationship with nonhuman entities, emphasizing reciprocity and respect for the natural world.

THE RELEVANCE OF CONNECTIVITY TO CULTURALLY COMPETENT NURSING

The diverse lenses provided earlier demonstrate how humans connect, relate to, and interact with other humans and inform healthcare providers about the significance of understanding and respecting the different worldviews for more effective connectivity. It is becoming more evident that the huge changes we witness in the 21st century not only require urgent consideration of our human lifestyles, needs, and behaviors but also equally require the inclusion of nonhuman entities and nature if we wish to live in an interconnected, healthier, happier, and more just world. Such an approach is very relevant to culturally competent care, which is currently human centered. This book encourages culturally competent health care providers to consider the benefits a more inclusive education and practice can bring to all people who need health and social care.

For example, educators can foster environmental and nonhuman health information in their human-centric, culturally competent curricula in the following ways:

- Learning native science and earth-based healing modalities (Cajete, 2000).
- Discussing medical technology's effects on care experiences (Latour, 2005).
- Fostering ethical reasoning on eco-justice impacts (Kimmerer, 2013).
- Appreciating people's spiritual connections to land and place (Kimmerer, 2013).
- Considering environmental and social factors' entwined effects on health (Ostrom, 2009).

Conclusion

This chapter defined and discussed six key concepts—communication, compassion, courage, collaboration, cybernetics, and connectivity—which are essential to the application of culturally competent and compassionate nursing and allied healthcare. The chapter provided meanings of the six concepts over different eras and contexts, from ancient to modern times and from different disciplines and perspectives, from philosophers to anthropologists, psychologists, political personalities, and AI and robotics theorists and practitioners. In our fast-changing world, nurses and other health professionals must acquire knowledge and skills that are broader than encompassed by today's nursing. It is imperative that a culturally competent and compassionate education include interdisciplinary learning. In order to understand the present and built skills for the future, the education of nurses and allied healthcare professionals must embrace the past. I liken this to the personal quest to understand one's roots, which will lead to personal enlightenment and guide one's current and future paths. In addition, conceptual frameworks illuminating human interconnectivity with nonhuman worlds and the environment provide invaluable insights into cultural competence. Exploring diverse cultural worldviews on nature fosters healthcare professionals' readiness to provide socially and ecologically conscious care.

According to Schwab (2016), the founder of the World Economic Forum, the Fourth Industrial Revolution begun at the turn of this century. It is changing how we live, work, and communicate. It is reshaping all aspects of government such as education, healthcare, and commerce. It will be changing our relationships, our opportunities, our identities, and even, in some cases, our bodies as it changes the physical and virtual worlds we inhabit. In the future, it can also change the things we value and the ways we value them. He urges all humans to work together and with nature and nonhuman entities in order to create a future for all, having fulfilling lives and helping the planet heal and remain the home of all entities living in harmony.

Activities

CRITIQUE (10 MINUTES)

Select one of the essential concepts in this chapter and try to critique it by asking questions, such as the following:

- *Is their explanation clear?*
- *Is it easy to understand or does it contain jargon or technical terms that need further explanation?*
- *Does it capture the essential elements and key aspects of the concept?*
- *Is the information provided about the concept factually correct and based on established theories or research?*
- *Does it avoid making broad generalizations or assumptions that may not apply in all contexts?*
- *Add your own questions.*

Record your opinions in your diary.

REFERENCES

Alizadeh, S., & Chavan, M. (2016). Cultural competence dimensions and outcomes: A systematic review of the literature. *Health and Social Care in the Community, 24*(6), e117–e130.

Aristotle. (1989). *Rhetoric*. Loeb Classic Library.

Aristotle. (2004). *Nicomachean ethics. Book II*. Penguin Classics.

Armstrong, K. (2011). *Twelve steps to a compassionate life*. Alfred A. Knopf.

Bakhtin, M. M. (1981). *The dialogic imagination: Four essays*. (M. Holquist, ed.; C. Emerson & M. Holquist, Trans.). University of Texas Press.

Banks, J. A., & McGee Banks, C. A. (Eds) (2019). *Multicultural Education: Issues and Perspectives*. 10th Edition. John Wiley & Sons, Inc.

Baumeister, R. F., & Leary, M. R. (1995). The need to belong: Desire for interpersonal attachments as a fundamental human motivation. *Psychological Bulletin, 117*(3), 497–529. https://doi.org/10.1037/0033-2909.117.3.497.

Braidotti, R. (2013). *The posthuman*. Polity Press.

Buber, M. (1970). *I and Thou*. (W. Kaufmann, Trans.). Charles Scribner's Sons.

Cajete, G. (2000). *Native science: Natural laws of interdependence*. Clear Light Publishers.

Capra, F., & Luisi, P. L. (2014). *The systems view of life: A unifying vision*. Cambridge University Press. https://doi.org/10.1017/CBO9780511895555.

Collins, F. S. (2003). The Human Genome Project: Lessons from large-scale biology. *Science, 300*(5617), 286–290.

Confucius (1979). In D. C. Lau (Ed.), *The Analects*. Penguin Books Trans.

D'Amour, D., Ferrada-Videla, M., San Martin Rodriguez, L., & Beaulieu, M. D. (2005). The conceptual basis for interprofessional collaboration: Core concepts and theoretical frameworks. *Journal of interprofessional care, 19*(sup1), 116–131.

Engster, D. (2007). *The heart of justice: Care ethics and political theory*. Oxford University Press.

Epicurus (Translated by E. O'Connor) (1993). *The essential Epicurus: Letters, principal doctrines, Vatican sayings, and fragments*. Prometheus Books.

Finney, B. (1976). Navigation. In E. S. Dodge (Ed.), *Islands and empires: Western impact on the pacific and East Asia. Europe and the world in age of expansion*, 8 (pp. 176–196). University of Minnesota Press.

Gandhi, M. K. (1913) Collected works. New Delhi, India. Publications Division, Ministry of Information and Broadcasting, Government of India 13 (pp. 241). Ch.153.

Goetz, J. L., Keltner, D., & Simon-Thomas, E. (2010). Compassion: An evolutionary analysis and empirical review. *Psychological Bulletin, 136*(3), 351–374. https://doi.org/10.1037/a0018807.

Grafman, J., & Krueger, F. (2009). The prefrontal cortex stores structured event complexes that are the representational basis for cognitively delivered actions. In E. Morsella, J. A. Bargh, & P. M. Gollwitzer (Eds.), *Oxford Handbook of human action*. Oxford University Press.

Greitemeyer, T., Fischer, P., Kastenmüller, A., & Frey, D. (2006). Civil courage and helping behavior: Differences and similarities. *European Psychologist, 11*(2), 90–98. https://doi.org/10.1027/1016-9040.11.2.90.

Guthrie, W. K. C. (1950). *The Greek philosophers from Thales to Aristotle*. Routledge.

Habermas, J. (1984). *The Theory of Communicative Action, Volume 1: Reason and the Rationalization of Society*. (T. McCarthy, Trans.). Beacon Press.

Habermas, J. (1987). *The Theory of Communicative Action, Volume 2: Lifeworld and System: A Critique of Functionalist Reason*. (T. McCarthy, Trans.). Beacon Press.

Hall, E. T. (1959). *The silent language*. Anchor.

Haraway, D. (2016). *Staying with the trouble*. Duke University Press.

Harbaugh, W. T., Mayr, U., & Burghart, D. R. (2007). Neural responses to taxation and voluntary giving reveal motives for charitable donations. *Science, 316*(5831), 1622–1625. https://doi.org/10.1126/science.1140738.

Heims, S. J. (1991). *The Cybernetics Group*. MIT Press.

Heuer, R. (2023). CERN's Accelerator Complex. Opening Lecture. CERN. https://home.cern/science/accelerators/cern-accelerator-complex.

International Space Station (ISS). (n.d.). https://en.wikipedia.org/wiki/International_Space_Station.

International Telecommunication Union (ITU). (2022). Global Connectivity Report 2022. Achieving universal and meaningful connectivity in the Decade of Action. Retrieved August 2023 from https://www.magonlinelibrary.com/doi/full/10.12968/bjmh.2020.0007.

Kidder, R. M. (2009). *Moral courage: Taking action when your values are put to the test*. HarperCollins.

Kimmerer, R. W. (2013). *Braiding sweetgrass: Indigenous wisdom, scientific knowledge and the teachings of plants* (Milkweed Editions).

Kirmayer, L. J. (2012). Cultural competence and evidence-based practice in mental health: epistemic communities and the politics of pluralism. *Social Science & Medicine, 75*(2), 249–256. https://doi.org/10.1016/j.socscimed.2012.03.018.

Kristjánsson, K. (2014). Is shame an ugly emotion? Four discourses—Two contrasting interpretations for moral education. *Studies in Philosophy and Education, 33*(5), 495–511. https://doi.org/10.1007/s11217-014-9417-4.

Latour, B. (2005). *Reassembling the social: An introduction to actor-network-theory*. Oxford University Press.

Low, K. C. P. (2011). Confucius, the value of benevolence and what's in it for humanity. *Conflict Resolution & Negotiation Journal, 2011*(1), 32–43.

Lyons, J. (2010). *The house of wisdom: How the Arabs transformed Western civilization*. Bloomsbury Publishing.

Macfarlane, J. (2020). Positive psychology: Social connectivity and its role within mental health nursing. *British Journal of Mental Health Nursing Practice, 9*(2). https://doi.org/10.12968/bjmh.2020.0007.

Mandela. (1994). *Long walk to freedom: The autobiography of Nelson Mandela*. Little, Brown.

Mark, J. J. (2017) The Egyptian Pyramids. *Ancient History Encyclopedia*. https://www.ancient.eu/Egyptian_Pyramids/

Mitchell, M. (2009). *Complexity: A guided tour*. Oxford University Press.

Moll, J., Krueger, F., Zahn, R., Pardini, M., de Oliveira-Souza, R., & Grafman, J. (2006). Human Fronto-mesolimbic networks guide decisions about charitable donation. *PNAS, 103*(42), 15623–15628. www.pnas.orgcgidoi. https://doi.org/10.1073/pnas.0604475103.

Morelli, S. A., Ong, D. C., Makati, R., Jackson, M. O., & Zaki, J. (2017). Empathy and well-being correlate with centrality in different social networks. In *Proceedings of the National Academy of Sciences of the United States of America*, 114, 9843–9847.

Murdoch, I. (1993). *Metaphysics as a guide to morals*. Penguin Books.

Murray, J. S. (2010). Moral courage in healthcare: Acting ethically even in the presence of risk. *The Online Journal of Issues in Nursing*. https://doi.org/10.3912/OJIN.Vol15No03Man02.

Neff, K. D. (2023). Self-compassion: Theory, method, research, and intervention. *Annual Review of Psychology, 74*, 193–217.

Neff et al. (n.d.). Publications by Kristin Neff and colleagues (in chronological order). Retrieved August 10, 2023, from https://self-compassion.org/wp-content/uploads/2023/05/SCPublicationsNeff_May2023.pdf/.

Nussbaum, M. C. (2001). *Upheavals of thought: The intelligence of emotions*. Cambridge University Press.

Oberauer, A.G. (2021). Posthumanism: A Philosophy for the 21st Century? Montreal, Canada: The Collector. https://www.thecollector.com/posthumanism-philosophy-of-the-21st-century/.)

Ostrom, E. (2009). A general framework for analysing sustainability of social-ecological systems. *Science, 325*(5939), 419–422.

Overbye, D. (2022). The LHC collider is back doing its universe-expanding thing. *The New York Times*.

Papadopoulos I. (2011). Courage, compassion and cultural competence. The 13th Anna Reynvaan Lecture. De Stadsschouwburg – Amsterdam City Theatre, the Netherlands.

Papadopoulos, I., Taylor, G., Ali, S., Aagard, M., Akman O., Alpers, L. M., ... Zorba A. (2017). Exploring nurses meaning and experiences of compassion: an international online survey involving 15 countries. *Journal of Transcultural Nursing, 28*(3), 286–295. https://doi.org/10.1177/1043659615624740.

Papadopoulos, I. (2018). *Culturally competent compassion: A guide for healthcare students and practitioners*. Routledge.

Papadopoulos, I., Zorba, A., Koulouglioti, C., Ali, S., Aagard, M., Akman, O., Alpers, L. M., Apostolara, P., Biles, J., Martín-García, Á., González-Gil, T., Kouta, C., Krepinska, R., Kumar, B. N., Lesińska-Sawicka, M., Lopez, L., Malliarou, M., Nagórska, M., Nissim, S., ... Vasiliou, M. (2016). International study on nurses' views and experiences of compassion. *International Nursing Review, 63*, 395–405.

Pavey, L., Greitemeyer, T., & Sparks, P. (2011). Highlighting relatedness promotes prosocial motives and behaviour. *Personality and Social Psychology Bulletin, 37*(7), 905–917. 2011. https://doi.org/10.1177/0146167211405994.

Pecukonis, E., Doyle, O., & Bliss, D. L. (2008). Reducing barriers to interprofessional training: Promoting interprofessional cultural competence. *Journal of Interprofessional Care, 22*(4), 417–428.

Pianalto, M. (2012). Moral courage and facing others. *International Journal of Philosophical Studies, 20*(2), 165–184.

Pickering, A. (2010). *The cybernetic brain: Sketches of another future*. University of Chicago Press.

Plato (1991). In A. Bloom (Ed.), *The Republic* (2nd ed.). Basic Books Trans.

Pury, C. S., Starkey, C. B., & Olson, L. R. (2023). Value of goal predicts accolade courage: more evidence that courage is a taking a *worthwhile* risk. *The Journal of Positive Psychology, 19*(2), 236–242. https://doi.org/10.1080/17439760.2023.2178959.

Putman, D. (1997). Psychological courage. *Philosophy, Psychiatry, & Psychology, 4*(1), 1–11. https://doi.org/10.1353/ppp.1997.0008.

Rizzolatti, G., & Fabbri-Destro, M. (2010). Mirror neurons: From discovery to autism. *Experimental Brain Research, 200*(3-4), 223–237. https://doi.org/10.1007/s00221-009-2002-3.

Saunders, J. (2015). Compassion. *Clinical Medicine, 1*(2), 121–124.

Schantz, M. L. (2007). Compassion: A concept analysis. *Nursing Forum, 42*(2), 48–55. https://doi.org/10.1111/j.1744-6198.2007.00067.x.

Scheman, N. (2011). *Shifting ground: Knowledge and reality, transgression and trustworthiness*. Oxford University Press.

Schwab, K. (2016). The fourth industrial revolution: What it means, how to respond. *World Economic Forum*. https://www.weforum.org/agenda/2016/01/the-fourth-industrial-revolution-what-it-means-and-how-to-respond/.

Spivak, G. C. (2010). *Can the subaltern speak? In Reflections on the history of an idea.* Columbia University Press.

Straughair, C. (2012). Exploring compassion. Implications for contemporary nursing. Part 1. *British Journal of Nursing, 21*(3), 160–164.

Taner, B. (n.d.). The role of resonant leadership in organisations. Retrieved August 10, 2023, from www.eujournal.org/index.php/esj/article/viewFile/1292/1301.

Taylor, C. (1991). *The ethics of authenticity.* Harvard University Press.

United Nations. (n.d.). https://www.un.org/en/about-us.

Watts, V. (2013). *Indigenous place-thought and agency amongst humans and non-humans (First Peoples, New Directions in Indigenous Studies).* University of Washington Press.

Wood, J. N., & Grafman, J. (2006). Human prefrontal cortex: Processing and representational perspectives. *Nature Reviews Neuroscience, 4*(2), 139–147.

Chapter 4

Culturally Competent and Virtuous Leadership

Learning Objectives

Upon completion of this chapter, readers should be able to:

- Gain knowledge of the notion of leadership in ancient and modern times.
- Raise their awareness of existing theories of leadership.
- Gain knowledge about the history and evolution of nursing leadership.
- Appreciate the desirability of culturally competent and virtuous leadership.
- List the components of culturally competent and virtuous leadership.
- Consider the consequences of 'bad' leadership.

Introduction

My work on leadership has been greatly influenced by the virtues of the Greek philosopher Aristotle (384–322 BC) and by the experiential and pragmatic approach of the late clinician and medical educator Dr. Aidan Halligan (1957–2015), who espoused that:

We know when we see a leader. They inspire us and when we're inspired we become determined. And when we are determined we go further. That's what leadership is about.... And it is your example that counts not you rank.

And if you care about patients to the point of being selfless, pleople will always respect that. (p. 80)

Halligan, 2014

In an increasingly interconnected world, culturally competent and virtuous leadership is emerging as an imperative skill set for individuals in positions of authority at the organizational, team, and individual levels. Effective leadership is no longer limited to traditional management skills; it must also encompass a deep understanding and appreciation of diverse cultures, backgrounds, and perspectives.

After a brief summary about the history of leadership, from ancient to contemporary eras, this chapter presents some historical and modern information about nursing leaders and leadership styles and achievements. The chapter goes on to argue that nursing and the health professions will benefit by adopting the culturally competent and virtuous leadership. This model of leadership is underpinned by the belief that nursing is an ethical activity and therefore should be founded on virtues, such as compassion, honesty, kindness, fairness, altruism, courage, forgiveness, and cooperation. In addition, nursing must cultivate the virtue of practical wisdom (phronesis), as this is the virtue by which all other virtues are given appropriate expression. Having explored the importance of culturally competent and virtuous leadership, the chapter highlights the toxic effects of non-virtuous leadership, especially in today's globalized societies.

Definitions

Leadership is the process of guiding, inspiring, and influencing individuals or groups to achieve common goals and objectives, often through effective communication, decision-making, and setting an example.

Cultural competence in leadership is the ability to navigate and thrive in multicultural environments, foster inclusivity, and leverage diversity to drive innovation and success.

Virtues are qualities or traits of moral excellence and ethical goodness, such as compassion, honesty, integrity, kindness, and courage, that guide and shape an individual's character and behavior in a positive and admirable way.

Many of the other Aristotelian virtues (Aristotle, 2004) were defined and described in the previous chapters.

1. **Phronesis (Practical wisdom):** Practical wisdom is the ability to make sound, morally informed decisions. In nursing leadership, this means applying cultural competence in decision-making. Leaders should have the wisdom to respect and consider cultural differences when crafting policies, protocols, and patient care plans.

2. **Courage (Andreia):** Courage is necessary to confront biases and stereotypes that may hinder culturally competent leadership. Leaders must have the courage to challenge discriminatory practices and promote cultural sensitivity within their teams.

3. **Compassion (Eleos):** Compassion is at the core of nursing leadership. A culturally competent leader shows empathy and concern for patients of all cultural backgrounds, ensuring their emotional and physical needs are met with sensitivity.

4. **Integrity (Arete):** Nursing leaders must exhibit moral integrity by adhering to principles of cultural competence, ensuring fair and equitable care for all patients, regardless of their cultural backgrounds.

5. **Generosity (Eucharistia):** Generosity involves sharing knowledge and resources. Culturally competent nursing leaders are generous in sharing best practices for delivering culturally sensitive care with their teams and supporting ongoing cultural competency training.

6. **Humility (Praotes):** Humility is essential in acknowledging one's own limitations and biases. Culturally competent nursing leaders recognize that they may not have all the answers and are open to learning from others, including their diverse staff and patients.

7. **Patience (Makrothymia):** Patience is vital when fostering a culture of cultural competence. Nursing leaders understand that it takes time for their teams to embrace these principles fully and for patients to feel comfortable expressing their cultural needs.

8. **Justice (Dikaiosune):** Justice in nursing leadership means ensuring equitable access to care, regardless of cultural differences. Culturally competent leaders

work to eliminate disparities and promote fairness in healthcare delivery.

9. **Empathy (*Sumpatheia*):** Empathy is the ability to understand and share the feelings of others. Nursing leaders, especially those focused on cultural competence, must demonstrate empathy to connect with patients from diverse backgrounds on a human level.

10. **Magnanimity (*Megalopsychia*):** Magnanimity involves greatness of soul, a willingness to do great things. In nursing leadership, this means aspiring to create an environment of inclusion and respect where every individual, regardless of their cultural background, can thrive.

Ancient and Modern Perspectives About Leadership

An article published on the Keele University's website in May 2023, titled "The History of Leadership", (University of Keele, 2023), highlighted the fact that human history is filled with leaders, from Alexander the Great to Abraham Lincoln, Mao Zedong, and Winston Churchill, and yet the concept of leadership is one that continues to inspire debate and study as people attempt to understand what leadership truly is. The chapter goes on to tell us that the use of the term "leadership" is thought to have originated in the 18th or 19th century, while the word "leader" was used as far back as the 14th century. However, the concept of leadership was present long before in ancient civilizations.

In the Far East, Confucianism promotes the view that the key virtue for leaders is *ren*—benevolence, humaneness, and love for others. According to his teachings, leaders should rule by moral example and seek to improve the lives of the people (Ames & Rosemont, 1998). Taoism promotes the notion that ideal leader should govern effortlessly through *wu-wei* or nonaction. These principles aligned with the natural order that lets things take their course without excessive control or forcing order (Watts & Huan, 1975). Buddhism teaches that leaders should rule with compassion, avoid harm, and seek enlightenment (Walshe, 2012).

In the West, the Greek philosopher Plato (428–348 BCE) argued that leaders should be philosopher-kings guided by wisdom and justice. Aristotle (384–322 BCE) argued that leaders should have practical wisdom and strong character virtues like courage, compassion, temperance, and justice (Ross & Brown, 2009; Aristotle, 1989). According to him, practical wisdom is the ability to do the right thing, at the right time, and for the right reasons.

In the early postmedieval era, the Italian political philosopher and statesman Niccolo Machiavelli (1469–1527) wrote his famous book, *The Prince*, in which he argued that leaders must be cunning and use power pragmatically. He prioritized order and control over virtue (Machiavelli, 1966).

Making a big leap forward, we find ourselves in the modern times of the 20th and 21st centuries. Building on the Eastern tradition of benevolence (Confucianism), the nonaction approach (Taoism), compassion (Buddhism), and Western thought from Greek virtue ethics (Aristotle) to pragmatic power (Machiavelli), modern theories of leadership emphasize representativeness, checks on power, and responsible leadership that serves the people's interests. Modern leadership also recognizes that a good leader can do the more difficult aspects of their role—making tough decisions, conducting evaluations, and so on—and also demonstrate humility, emotional intelligence, and flexibility.

The summary in Table 4.1 provides information about the most commonly cited modern theories of leadership. The reader may build the path of the evolution of leadership influenced by ancient theories, time, and societal changes.

Leadership in Healthcare: The Modern Era

Before we explore the "Papadopoulos model of culturally competent and virtuous nursing leadership," let us briefly consider the recent developments in healthcare leadership from some of the UK leading institutions.

To begin with, in 2011, The King's Fund published a report, titled *The future of leadership and management in the NHS: No more heroes report* (The King's Fund, 2011), which defined leadership as the art of motivating a group of people to achieve a common goal. This was followed by two other publications

in 2015. The National Centre for Ethics in Health Care report (Cook et al., 2015) states that a key responsibility in leadership is ensuring that the organization encourages employees to "do the right thing." As such, leaders should foster an environment and an organizational culture that support doing the right thing and doing it well, for reasons that are supported by ethical values. This statement is obviously based on the Aristotelian ethics.

Meanwhile, the Faculty of Medical Leadership and Management (FMLM), The King's Fund, and the Center for Creative Leadership (CCL) (West et al., 2015) collectively initiated a review of the evidence for leadership, the findings of which are summarized as follows:

- Leadership is required to ensure the delivery of high-quality and compassionate patient care.
- Leadership is required to develop inspiring visions operationalized at every level.
- Leadership is required to embody support for staff, honesty, kindness, altruism, fairness, accountability, and optimism.
- Leadership is required to ensure cultures that are not preoccupied with target

TABLE 4.1 The Evolution of Leadership Theories in the Modern Era		
Author's Name Birth and Death Dates	**Name of Theory and Dates of Development**	**Key Concepts and Principles of Theories**
Thomas Carlyle (1795–1881)	Great Man theory 1840s	• Leaders arise when there is a need for their talents and skills. • Leaders are born with innate traits and abilities destined to rise and lead. • Theory focused entirely on males and masculine stereotypes.
Kurt Lewin (1890–1947)	Theory of three leadership styles 1939	• This theory determined that there were three basic leadership styles: Authoritarian (Autocratic), Participative (Democratic), and Delegative (Laissez-Faire).

Continued on following page

TABLE 4.1 **The Evolution of Leadership Theories in the Modern Era** (Continued)		
Author's Name **Birth and Death Dates**	**Name of Theory and** **Dates of Development**	**Key Concepts and Principles of Theories**
Ralph Melvin Stogdill (1905–1978)	Trait theory 1948	• People with certain innate traits are more likely to attain leadership positions. • Important leadership traits are intelligence, initiative, persistence, self-confidence, sociability, and responsibility.

Ralph Stogdill
  (1904–1978)
John Hemphill
  (1919–1983)
Alvis Coons (B & D dates
  not known)
Rensis Likert
  (1903–1981)
	Behavioral Late
	1940s–1950s
		• Effective leadership depends on the appropriate mix and display of task-focused and person-focused behaviors.
		• Employee-centered vs production-centered behaviors.
		• Leaders can be trained to exhibit these behaviors to improve leadership effectiveness rather than relying on inherited traits.

Fred Fiedler (1922–2017)	Contingency 1960	• Leadership effectiveness depends on the interaction between leadership style and situational factors. • This theory introduced the concept of "situational contingency," arguing there is no single best style of leadership. • Leaders must look beyond universal styles and recognize the impact of contexts.

Paul Hersey (1932–2021)
  and Ken Blanchard
  (1939)
	Situational 1969	• Focused more directly on the behaviors that leaders should adopt in specific situations.
		• Includes four leadership styles—telling, selling, participating, and delegating—based on directive and supportive behaviors.
		• Leaders need flexibility to diagnose situations and choose appropriate behaviors.

James MacGregor Burns (1918–2014)	Transactional 1978	• Transactional leadership involves exchanges or "transactions" between leaders and followers. • Leaders provide rewards or disciplinary action to motivate desired performance and obedience from followers.
James MacGregor Burns (1918–2014)	Transformational 1978	• Transformational leadership aims to motivate and inspire followers to achieve goals and create meaningful change. • Transformational leaders appeal to ideals and ethics to elevate followers' goals and inspire change. • Some key aspects of transformational leadership include charisma, inspiration, intellectual stimulation, and individualized consideration of followers' needs and motivations.

setting, rules, regulations, and status hierarchies.

- Leadership is most effective when all staff accept responsibility for their leadership roles, especially doctors, nurses, and other clinicians.
- Leadership requires leaders to work together, spanning organizational boundaries both within and between organizations, prioritizing overall patient care, and working collectively to build a cooperative, integrative collective leadership culture.
- Experience in leadership is the most valuable factor in enabling leaders to develop their skills, especially when they have appropriate guidance and support. Focusing on how to enhance leaders' learning from experience should be a priority.
- National level leadership is required to ensure the overarching national organizations (Monitor, CQC, NHS England, NHS Trust Development Authority) exemplify models of collective leadership, positive cultures, and have a core orientation of compassion toward the entire health service.

The aforementioned recommendations illustrate the importance of understanding the ancient leadership pronouncements and the relatively modern theories of leadership, which function as examples to build on their wise and beneficial contributions, while leaving behind those with negative approaches. The world is changing constantly, and new ideas or recycled beneficial ones need to be developed and implemented, taking into consideration the changes in time, sociocultural norms, medical interventions, and public demands and needs.

A Brief History of the Evolution of Nursing Leadership in Different Eras

In ancient Greece, the famous physician Hippocrates, who lived around 400 BCE, was credited with elevating medicine from a sacred art to a rational science. Under his influence, medicine and nursing became more professionalized and separated from the temple.

In ancient Roman times, wealthy Roman households often had slaves trained in medicine and nursing to care for the health needs of the family.

In India, the earliest hospitals were established by Buddhist monks around 230 BCE. The monks provided care to the sick and poor. Hindu scriptures also describe the role of women caregivers who assisted during childbirth and recovery. However, formal nursing as a profession did not emerge until much later.

The early Christian period saw the emergence of organized nursing care in some regions. Christian emphasis on charity led to the creation of small hospitals staffed by religious nursing orders and congregations of men and women.

Much later—in the 19th century—nursing began to establish itself as a unique profession.

The British nursing pioneer Florence Nightingale (1820–1910) established the world's first nursing school in 1860 at St. Thomas's Hospital in London. Her endeavors professionalized nursing through advocacy, training, and statistics. Her leadership principles focused on hygiene, order, and discipline.

Another pioneer of that era was the Jamaican Mary Seacole (1805–81), who, like

Nightingale, nursed wounded soldiers in the Crimean war. She is credited with adaptability and resourceful leadership style.

In 1899, the International Council of Nurses (ICN) was established. Over the years, the ICN has made significant achievements in advancing the nursing profession and improving global health. In 1996, the ICN established the Leadership for Change programme and the Global Nursing Leadership Institute in 2008 to develop and strengthen nursing leadership worldwide.

In the post-Nightingale era (1900s–1920s), the American nurse leaders Linda Richards and Lavinia Dock established training schools and pushed for nurse licensing.

During the World War II era (1940s), nurse leaders emerged having direct authority in military-style hierarchy. In the post–World War II era (1950s–1960s), nurse leaders adopted—as many other disciplines did at the time—the bureaucratic, centralized authority styles. The modern era (1970s–present) finds nurses and nurse leaders gaining access to higher education. Leadership has been evolving, embracing emerging styles like transformational servant leadership to empower nurses.

Genesis and Evolution of Culturally Competent Leadership in Nursing

In the early history of nursing, cultural awareness was minimal. Mabel Keaton Staupers (1890–1989) was an influential leader in the American Nurses Association. She fought for equal opportunities for Black nurses and successfully pushed for the admission of Black nurses into the American Red Cross during World War II. Estelle Massey Osborne (1901–1981), the first African American nurse to earn a master's degree in the United States in 1946, advocated for more education opportunities for Black nurses. She served as the first Black president of the American Nurses Association from 1970 to 1972. Both Osborne and Staupers spoke out against discrimination in the nursing profession and in nursing education. They pushed for policies and programs to increase minority representation and provide equal opportunities for all nurses. Their advocacy work increased awareness of the needs and challenges faced by minority nurses. They paved the way for more inclusive policies and diversification of the nursing workforce. They highlighted the importance of considering culture in providing care to diverse patient populations.

During the 1950s–1980s, nursing leaders pushed for more inclusion and antidiscrimination practices. Multiculturalism motivated nurse leaders to promote cultural awareness as demographics diversified. Transcultural nursing (the antecedent of cultural competence) had arrived via the work of Madeleine Leininger (1925–2012), who highlighted the importance of gaining cultural knowledge in order to provide effective care to people of different cultural backgrounds. During the 1990s–2000s, nurse leaders became more aware of cultural competence, the need for it, and its benefits. In some countries, cultural competence was embraced by educators, researchers, and practice leaders. Since the 2000s, more attention is given by nurse leaders to global health disparities and migration. The concepts of cultural humility and cultural intelligence were also introduced in research and education as complementary to the existing concepts. Recently, leadership styles are emphasizing advocacy, compassion, responsiveness to communities, and health equity.

Why Culturally Competent Virtuous Leadership?

Sellman (2011) suggests that *"nursing is an inherently moral practice and that this places moral obligations on individual nurses to cultivate the sorts of dispositions necessary to ensure that nursing actions enable rather than diminish human flourishing"* (pp. 17–18).

As a practice-oriented profession, nursing must cultivate the virtue of practical wisdom (phronesis)—which was mentioned in an earlier section of this chapter—as this is the virtue by which all other virtues are given appropriate expression. According to Aristotle, practical wisdom is the ability to do the right thing at the right time and for the right reasons.

In considering the nature of moral and ethical leadership in nursing, Gallagher and Tschudin (2010) argued that all members of the nursing workforce are ethical leaders insofar as they demonstrate a commitment to ethical practice in their everyday work and act as ethical role models for others. Nurse leaders are responsible for influencing their teams and for acting as arbiters between organizational and professional values.

Goode and Like (2012) argued that strong and informed nursing leadership is required in order to achieving patient services that are culturally and linguistically competent. They recommend that leadership should ensure that:

- Cultural and linguistic competence is cultivated at all levels of healthcare organizations and systems.
- The role of a nursing leader must be revisited and adapted to address ongoing and emerging challenges such as organizational change processes, differences across and within cultures, and resulting dynamics, resistance, and power differentials.

During the last decade of the 20th century and the first (almost) three decades of the 21st century, a significant number of nursing and midwifery leadership failures were reported. For example:

1. Beverley Allitt (1991)—An English pediatric nurse who murdered four children and injured nine others with high doses of insulin while working at a hospital. She is known as the "Angel of Death."
2. Mid Staffordshire NHS Trust scandal (2009–2013)—Reports of neglect and mistreatment of patients at Stafford Hospital in England led to public inquiries revealing severe failings in nursing care and leadership.
3. Victorino Chua (2015)—A Filipino nurse convicted in the United Kingdom of murdering 2 patients and poisoning 20 others at a hospital. He contaminated saline bags with insulin.
4. Lucy Letby (2015–2016) was a British nurse who had been convicted of murdering 5 babies and attempting to murder 10 others while working in the neonatal unit of the Countess of Chester Hospital.

These shocking cases gained significant media attention and damaged public perception of nursing and midwifery. However, these are rare instances that do not represent the dedicated care provided by most nurses and midwives. These cases raised difficult questions about leadership, security, and organizational cultures.

Although the aforementioned cases are rare, we must acknowledge that a huge number of "near misses" or "no harm events" are reported each year in the United Kingdom. The NHS England defines a near miss as a "prevented patient safety incident which although did not cause harm, it has the potential to cause injury or ill health." The following numbers are from all health professions including the nursing profession, which has the biggest number of care providers in each healthcare institution.

- The NHS estimates over 700,000 incidents are reported through its National Reporting and Learning System (NRLS) each year. This system collects reports of patient safety incidents from healthcare organizations.
- Not all of these qualify as true "near misses" or "no harm events". But data indicate that around 9000 reports per month are classified as no harm incidents.
- Extrapolating from this, we can estimate that over 100,000 "no harm events" or near misses are reported per year through the NRLS.
- The NRLS is voluntary and so may underrepresent the true number. Other studies estimate the true number could be over three times higher when including unreported events.

Each of the reported near misses will have its own story. But ultimately, when a patient's safety is compromised, his/her care was insufficient, wrongly provided by staff lacking the relevant knowledge and skills, a working environment lacking in moral principles and virtues leading to inhumane and negligent practices, poor communication between the staff and patients, lack of cultural competence, and poor leadership.

What Are the Components of Culturally Competent and Virtuous Leadership?

Dr. Aidan Halligan (1957–2015) espoused that "*At its core, leadership is a purely moral and emotional activity. It is unconnected with seniority and only loosely related to intellect and it is about the ability to engage, motivate and inspire. It is defined by our values and implies having moral courage, integrity and the conviction to accept accountability*" (Halligan, 2014 p. 82). Wise words, highlighting the connection between practical wisdom and genuine interest for our fellow humans, to that of leadership. It could be argued that the pragmatism in Halligan's explanation of leadership has been based on his vast experience as a clinician and medical educator, while his emphasis on virtues was influenced by classical philosophies that are still used today, such as the philosophy of Aristotle.

The key components of the Papadopoulos model of leadership, which I have called *culturally competent and virtuous leadership*, are based on the four constructs I used for the creation of my model for cultural competence (Papadopoulos, 2006): cultural awareness, cultural knowledge, cultural sensitivity, and cultural competence. The model is fully explained in Chapter 2 of this book.

The key virtues used—compassion, courage, genuine friendship, proper self-love, and forgiveness—originate from Aristotle. At the beginning of this chapter, I provided the following definition of virtues: *Virtues are qualities or traits of moral excellence and ethical goodness, such as compassion, honesty, integrity, kindness, and courage, that guide and shape an individual's character and behavior in a positive and admirable way.* According to Aristotle, a virtue lies between two vices. For example,

TABLE 4.2 The Toxic Vices of Leadership	
Toxic Effects of Leadership Based on Extreme Collectivism	**Toxic Effects of Leadership Based on Extreme Self-interest/Individualism**
• Codependence and co-collusion • Group-think • Lack of whistleblowers • In-group conformity pressure • Exploitative, excessive interest in each other • Lack of personal growth and low levels of self-awareness • Lack of self-leadership • Suppression of dissent and diverse opinions • Tolerance of poor standards of care	• Self-interest-driven action • Lack of interest in each other as people • Exploitative behaviors • Competitiveness • Lack of trust • Lack of belongingness • Psychological insecurity • Destructive conflict • Energy draining and burnout

the virtue of courage lies between the vices of rashness and cowardice. The coward has too much fear, which leads to inability to act or acting inappropriately; the rash person has too little fear and excessive confidence, which may also lead to inappropriate or even harmful acts to the self and/or the person/purpose for whom/which the courage is directed. The courageous person has the right amount of fear to be able to overcome it.

I propose that culturally competent and virtuous leadership lies between the vices of extreme collectivism and extreme self-interest/individualism. Leadership at either end of the leadership pole is toxic and can have catastrophic results, as many of the recent reports attest. Table 4.2 provides some suggestions of the toxic vices of leadership that may lie at the extreme ends of the leadership continuum.

In between the two toxic vices lie the components of the culturally competent and virtuous leadership's golden mean depicted as the arrow of practical wisdom (phronesis) in Figure 4.1.

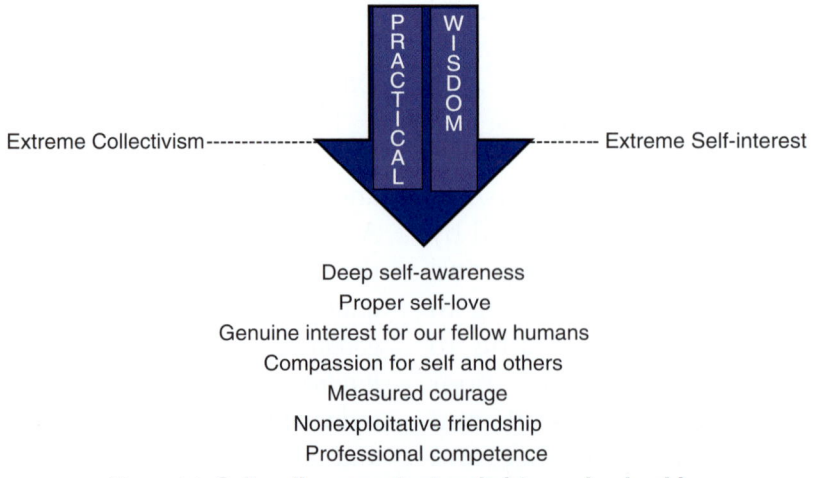

Extreme Collectivism-------------- PRACTICAL WISDOM --------- Extreme Self-interest

Deep self-awareness
Proper self-love
Genuine interest for our fellow humans
Compassion for self and others
Measured courage
Nonexploitative friendship
Professional competence

Figure 4.1 Culturally competent and virtuous leadership.

A culturally competent and virtuous leader is one who possesses deep self-awareness. An awareness of one's own cultural values and identity and the need for self-compassion is fundamental for a leader who wishes to inspire those they are working with. Crucial to this is the attainment of the virtue of proper self-love and self-knowledge (aftognosia), which guides our actions toward understanding, caring, and respecting our self. It is important for leaders to understand that their self is not complete without a relationship with the selves of those they lead and who may come from a variety of cultural backgrounds; therefore, equal amounts of culturally competent understanding, caring, and respect must be given to them. The friendships of this leader are genuine channels of intercultural communication and a healthy interest for the person behind the professional worker. In nurturing a virtuous working environment, this leader, through his/her own behavior and culturally competent acts, is a compassionate role model who understands the emotional suffering of his/her coworkers and sensitively responds to them. Within this approach, leaders do not form friendships in order to exploit them for self-gain (such as self-advancement). Diversity is celebrated, and the leader encourages staff to engage with it by providing co-learning opportunities. Openness and freedom to express views related to the improvement of the quality of services offered to patients are paramount. But even in such caring and democratic working environments, the enactment of measured courage must be nurtured. Small and medium-sized teams operate within larger organizations that continuously evolve to respond to changes to national policy, in the population, science and technology, economy, politics, and so on. Not every change is consulted upon and not every change results in improvements. These are some of the factors the culturally competent and virtuous leader considers seriously by asking:

- Are these the right changes, is this the right time for them, and are they required for the right reasons?
- Do I have adequate understanding as to the effects of these changes on our work, and if not, what resources should I be providing for my team?
- How do I empower my team to have the courage to challenge changes that will not contribute to the flourishing of the patients, staff, and organization?
- What strategies should I be putting in place to help the team deal with the consequences of their speaking up?
- Am I able to provide culturally competent and compassionate support to my multicultural team when dealing with ethical dilemmas?

Apart from inspiring, supporting, and empowering others, a leader is without a doubt the guardian of quality and standards. He/she has the responsibility, in collaboration with colleagues at different levels of the organization, to promote high-quality service provision that is culturally and compassionately competent and which strives to eliminate health inequalities. This means that the professional competencies of all staff members have to be kept updated and enhanced to cope with the ever-growing complexity of clinical practice in multicultural environments. Equally important is his/her contribution toward nurturing high-quality working environments and championing employment standards that promote equal opportunities and human flourishing.

In an international survey that I recently led (Papadopoulos et al., 2021), the virtue of compassion, one of the five Aristotelian key virtues, was explored with nursing and midwifery leaders. The study, which included 17 countries and 1217 participants in leadership positions, aimed to collect their views on the following three questions: (1) "How do you define compassion?" (2) "Can you list the advantages of giving compassion to staff?" and (3) "Can you explain why receiving compassion is important to you?"

Managers/leaders from all the participating countries defined compassion in terms of humanness, speaking to the universal dimension of compassion. The relationship between humane and compassionate healthcare that the participants expressed parallels conceptions put forward by the academic community (Crowther et al., 2013; Papadopoulos, 2018). Managers/leaders from South America and the Philippines—two collectivist cultures where in-group cohesion and a sense of a shared humanity appear higher (Oyserman et al., 2002)—overwhelmingly emphasized how compassion pertains to the essence of being human. The attention to a humane approach was expressed by Central–Eastern European managers/leaders, against the backdrop of the radical set of reforms in postcommunist health transitions (Safaei, 2012). These reforms had led to uncertainty in the workplace (Bludau, 2014), thus motivating healthcare leaders—including nurse leaders—to embrace the virtuous approach that emphasizes compassion, courage, non-exploitative friendship, and forgiveness.

Compassion was seen as a factor in establishing a trustworthy manager/leader–staff relationship, which was prevalent in the United States. The United States is a predominantly individualistic country, and it is widely accepted that employers focus on productivity and fear of litigation. These factors may explain managers/leaders' desire to establish relationships with their staff informed by trust and honesty. Other participants conflated compassion with sadness and pity (which may or may not lead to supportive action). This definition of compassion emerged in countries where traditional Christian Catholic values (e.g., Italy, Spain, and Colombia) are more strongly held.

The findings revealed that the benefits of compassionate leadership could be viewed as a continuum. At one end is the emphasis on the self (the manager/leader), moving through the benefits of compassion for the manager/leader–staff relationship, staff well-being, and teamwork, and, finally, at the other end, are the broader benefits for the work setting.

Finally, our evidence highlighted the crucial role of managers/leaders in establishing culturally competent and compassionate workplace cultures, which undoubtedly can influence the quality of patient care (Beardsmore & McSherry, 2017). Some of the culturally competent components and manifestations of compassion offered by the study's participants echo the compassion components reported by practicing nurses in another study, such as giving time, being there, defending and advocating, and personalization (Papadopoulos et al., 2016, 2017). This suggests that compassion giving is not drastically affected by the position one occupies in an organization.

Compassion in management/leadership is increasingly recognized as a "transcultural source of wisdom" (Opdebeeck & Habisch, 2011). Kleinman (2015) pointed out that "caregiving is relational and reciprocal" and can be conceived anthropologically as a "gift exchange," which is "moral, emotional, and practical" (p. 240). Our findings suggest that compassion giving and receiving form a symbiotic transactional relationship because a compassion giver always receives some compassion back, directly from the receiver or indirectly as self-growth, which may or may not be recognized immediately. Therefore, if compassion in general is viewed as a transactional act, it means that culturally situated transactional compassion can be a beneficial and potent tool to transcend otherness, and ensure authentic caregiving, at all levels of the organization. The majority of the nursing and midwifery managers/leaders participating in this study expressed how compassion relates to the establishment of caring relationships that bear emotional investment and cultural resonance (Jones, 2005), as well as compassionate workplaces characterized by a focus on care, instead of productivity, and by flourishing relationships and collaborations. Transactional culturally competent compassion—as a quintessential nursing quality—should sit at the core of nursing leadership.

The Papadopoulos Principles of Culturally Competent and Virtuous Nursing Leadership

Table 4.3 provides some key principles for culturally competent and virtuous leadership in nursing.

Posthumanism and Culturally Competent and Virtuous Nursing Leadership

In Chapter 1, I introduced the posthumanist theory and its relation to culture; in Chapter 2, we examined the meaning of E.M.B.R.A.C.E.

TABLE 4.3 Key Principles for Culturally Competent and Virtuous Leadership in Nursing	
Cultural awareness	Self-examination of one's own cultural identity, values, biases, and how these influence perceptions of others.
Cultural knowledge	Learning about the cultural beliefs, values, practices, history, and context of different groups.
Cultural sensitivity	Interacting respectfully through verbal and nonverbal communication tailored to cultural norms.
Cultural competence	Applying knowledge and sensitivity to provide optimal culturally appropriate care, mentoring students and colleagues, and championing equality, diversity, and inclusivity.
Cultural humility	Lifelong critical self-reflection and commitment to understanding diverse worldviews.
Virtuous leadership	Leading by example through ethical and virtuous behaviors such as being compassionate, courageous, honest, kind, friendly, considerate, respectful, etc.
Holistic care	Considering psychological, social, spiritual, biological, and environmental dimensions.
Patient/family-centred	Partnering with and empowering patients/families in care decisions.
Respecting nonhuman entities and the environment	Embracing the interconnectedness of all beings, both human and nonhuman, and the environment, recognizing their inherent value and contributions to health and nursing.

from the posthumanist lens; in Chapter 3, we explored the contribution of the posthumanist theory to culturally competent communication and the notion of connectivity from the posthumanist perspective.

Let us now consider briefly the relation of posthumanism to culturally competent and virtuous nursing leadership. To begin with, my culturally competent and virtuous nursing leadership theory is modeled on the Aristotelian ethical virtues like compassion, courage, and integrity, while the posthumanist theory incorporates similar values such as social justice, sustainability, and interconnected well-being. Both theories promote inclusivity and diversity. Nursing leadership emphasizes understanding and respecting the diverse cultural backgrounds and beliefs of patients. Posthumanism aligns with this by advocating for an inclusive approach that recognizes the multiplicity of human experiences, including cultural and technological. Furthermore, the posthumanist principles of pluralism, diversity, and contextual interpretation of reality resonate with cultural competence's aim to provide care tailored to patients' varied cultural identities, norms, and meanings. Technological advances in healthcare compel nursing leaders to reconsider human–technology relations. Virtuous nursing leadership involves making ethically sound decisions that prioritize patient well-being and justice. Posthumanism raises ethical questions related to the integration of technology into healthcare and the potential impact on human identity. Both posthumanism and culturally competent and virtuous nursing leadership call for adaptability. Nursing leaders need to be flexible in their approaches, understanding that healthcare is continuously evolving with the introduction of new technologies. Virtuous nursing leadership includes empowering patients to make informed decisions about their healthcare. Posthumanism, in a similar vein, highlights the importance of patient autonomy in an era where technology can both support and challenge traditional healthcare norms. Culturally competent and virtuous nursing leaders need to encourage their teams to stay updated on cultural competence and technological advancements to provide the best care.

Conclusion

The challenges of developing and adopting culturally competent and compassionate/virtuous leaders and leadership must not be underestimated. To ignore them would be a disastrous mistake, as ineffective leadership that lacks compassion can be dehumanizing to patients and staff alike. This chapter explored and discussed the importance of culturally competent and virtuous nursing leadership, which can have a profound connection to happiness, both for healthcare professionals and for the patients they serve, as it creates an environment where patients receive better care, healthcare professionals feel valued and empowered, and health disparities are reduced. This, in turn, fosters happiness among both patients and healthcare providers, as they experience improved well-being, job satisfaction, and a sense of fulfilment in contributing to positive health outcomes and societal progress.

Key Points About Nursing and Healthcare Leadership

- Effective leadership is no longer limited to traditional management skills; it must also encompass a deep understanding and appreciation of diverse cultures, backgrounds, and perspectives.

- The complexities of multicultural societies and the growing health inequalities require nursing and other health professions to have culturally competent and virtuous leadership.
- Culturally competent and virtuous leadership is an ethical activity founded on virtues such as compassion, honesty, kindness, fairness, altruism, and cooperation.
- Nursing must cultivate the virtue of practical wisdom (phronesis), as this is the virtue by which all other virtues (those of the intellect and of the character) are given appropriate expression.
- According to Aristotle, practical wisdom is the ability to do the right thing at the right time and for the right reasons.
- Nonvirtuous leadership can be toxic for individuals and the collective.
- Culturally competent and virtuous nursing leaders need to encourage their teams to stay updated on cultural competence and technological advancements to provide the best care.

Aristotle proffered that the purpose of living is to achieve happiness (*Eudaimonia*), which he called the "chief good." And how did he propose we achieve this? By living a virtuous life!

Activity

Access the report of the IENE4 leadership model and learning tools at:

http://ieneproject.eu/download/Outputs/Report_of_the_tools.PDF

Browse through the report to discover how the leadership model was developed and validated and how the learning units associated with the model were developed and evaluated. Select from the range of learning tools included in the report the one most relevant to your work. Read it and write a short reflective account on how informative and useful the tool was.

REFERENCES

Ames, R. T., & Rosemont, H. (1998). *The Analects of Confucius: A Philosophical Translation*. Ballantine Books.

Aristotle. (1989). *Rhetoric*. Loeb Classic Library.

Aristotle. (2004). *Nicomachean Ethics. Book II*. Penguin Classics.

Aristotle, (contributors: Ross W.D., Brown L.). (2009). *The Nicomachean Ethics*. Oxford University Press.

Beardsmore, E., & McSherry, R. (2017). Healthcare workers' perceptions of organisational culture and the impact on the delivery of compassionate quality care. *Journal of Research in Nursing, 22*(1-2), 42–56. https://doi.org/10.1177/1744987116685594.

Bludau, H. (2014). The power of protocol: Professional identity development and governmentality in post-socialist health care. *Sociologický Časopis/Czech Sociological, Časopis/Czech Sociological Review, 50*(6), 875–896. https://doi.org/10.13060/00380288.2014.50.6.145.

Burns, J. M. (1978). *Leadership*. New York: Harper & Row.

Carlyle, T. (1841). *On heroes, hero-worship, and the heroic in history*. James Fraser.

Cook, R., Foglia, M. B., Landon, M. K, & Bottrell, M. M. (2015). *Preventive Ethics: Addressing Ethics Quality Gaps on a Systems Level* (2nd ed.). U.S. Department of Veterans Affairs; National Center for Ethics in Health Care. (Retrieved from,. https://www.ethics.va.gov/docs/integratedethics/pe_primer_2_edition_042015.pdf).

Crowther, J., Wilson, K. C., Horton, S., & Lloyd-Williams, M. (2013). Compassion in healthcare: Lessons from a qualitative study of the end of life care of people with dementia. *Journal of the Royal Society of Medicine, 106*(12), 492–497. https://doi.org/10.1177/0141076813503593.

Fiedler, F. (1964). A Contingency Model of Leadership Effectiveness. In: Berkowitz, L. (Ed.), A Contingency Model of Leadership Effectiveness. *Advances in Experimental Social Psychology, 1*, 149–190. https://doi.org/10.1016/S0065-2601(08)60051-9.

Gallagher, A., & Tschudin, V. (2010). Educating for ethical leadership. *Nurse Education Today, 30*(3), 224–227.

Goode, T. D., & Like, R. C. (2012). Advancing and sustaining cultural and linguistic competence in the American health system: challenges, strategies, and lessons learned. In D. Ingleby, A. Chiarenza, W. Deville, & I. Kotsioni (Eds.), *Inequalities in health care for Migrants and Ethnic Minorities*, 2. Garant Publishers COST series on Health and Diversity.

Halligan, A. (2014). *Learning Leadership: How to become a leader in the NHS. (YouTube video no longer available)* Cited by Papadopoulos I. (2018). *Culturally competent compassion. A guide for healthcare students and practitioners*. (pp. 80–82). Routledge.

Hemphill, J. K., & Coons, A. E. (1957). Development of the Leader Behaviour Description Questionnaire. In R. M. Stogdill, & A. E. Coons (Eds.), *Leader behaviour: Its description and measurement* (pp. 6–38). Ohio State University, Bureau of Business Research.

Hersey, P., & Blanchard, K. H. (1969). Life Cycle Theory of Leadership. *Training Development, 23*, 26–34.

Jones, A. M. (2005). The anthropology of leadership: Culture and corporate leadership in the American South. *Leadership, 1*(3), 259–278. https://doi.org/10.1177/1742715005054437.

The King's Fund. (2011). *The Future of leadership and Management in the NHS. No more heroes. Report from The King's Fund Commission on Leadership and Management in the NHS*. The King's Fund.

Kleinman, A. (2015). Care: In search of a health agenda. *Lancet, 386*(9990), 240–241. https://doi.org/10.1016/S0140-6736(15). 61271-5.

Lewin, K., Lippitt, R., & White, R. K. (1939). Patterns of aggressive behaviour in experimentally created "social climates. *The Journal of Social Psychology, 10*(2), 269–299.

Likert, R. (1961). *New patterns of management*. McGraw-Hill.

Machiavelli, N. (1966). *The Prince*. University of America Press.

Opdebeeck, H., & Habisch, A. (2011). Compassion: Chinese and western perspectives on practical wisdom in management. *Journal of Management Development, 30*(7/8), 778–788. https://doi.org/10.1108/02621711111150272.

Oyserman, D., Coon, H. M., & Kemmelmeier, M. (2002). Rethinking individualism and collectivism: Evaluation of theoretical assumptions and meta-analyses. *Psychological Bulletin, 128*(1), 3–72. https://doi.org/10.1037/0033-2909.128.1.3.

Papadopoulos, I. (Ed.). (2006). *Transcultural Health and Social Care: Development of Culturally Competent Practitioners*. Churchill Livingstone, Elsevier.

Papadopoulos I., Wright S., Lazzarino R., et al. (2021). Enactment of compassionate leadership by nursing and midwifery managers: results from an international online survey. *BMJ Leader*, Published Online First: 27 September 2021. doi:10.1136/leader-2020-000385.

Papadopoulos, I, et al. (2021). The importance of being a compassionate leader: The views of nursing and midwifery managers from around the world. *Journal of Transcultural Nursing*, 1–13. https://doi.org/10.1177/10436596211008214.

Papadopoulos, I., et al. (2016). International study on nurses' views and experiences of compassion. *International Nursing Review, 63*, 395–405.

Papadopoulos, I., et al. (2017). Exploring nurses meaning and experiences of compassion: An international online survey involving 15 countries. *Journal of Transcultural Nursing, 28*(3), 286–295.

Papadopoulos, I. (2018). *Culturally competent compassion*. Routledge.

Plato. (1991). *The Republic*. Basic Books.

Safaei, J. (2012). Post-communist health transitions in Central and Eastern Europe. *Economics Research International, 2012*, 137412. https://doi.org/10.1155/2012/137412.

Sellman, D. (2011). *What Makes a Good Nurse*. Jessica Kingsley Publishers.

Stogdill, R. M. (1948). Personal factors associated with leadership: A survey of the literature. *The Journal of Psychology, 25*(1), 35–71. doi:10.1080/00223980.1948.9917362.

University of Keele. (2023). *The history of leadership*. Posted on: May 16, 2023 Retrieved from. https://online.keele.ac.uk/the-history-of-leadership/#:~:text=The%20first%20theory%20on%20leadership,even%20divine%20or%20fated%20destinies.

Walshe, M. (2012). *The Long Discourses of the Buddha: A Translation of the Digha Nikaya*. Wisdom Publications.

Watts, A., & Huan, A. (1975). *Tao: The Watercourse Way*. Pantheon.

West, M., Armit, K., Loewenthal, L., Eckert, R., West, T., & Lee, A. (2015). *Leadership Development in Health Care: The Evidence Base*. The Faculty of Medical Leadership and Management with The King's Fund and the Center for Creative Leadership.

Chapter 5

Culturally Competent and Compassionate Spiritual Care: Lessons From the COVID-19 Pandemic

Learning Objectives

After reading this chapter, you should:

- Become familiar with essential definitions relevant to this chapter.
- Become aware of major health disasters (MHDs) of the 20th and 21st centuries.
- Gain a deep appreciation of the physical, psychological, and moral challenges faced by the nursing workforce during the COVID-19 pandemic.
- Gain knowledge about the spiritual care (SC) rituals for death and dying of diverse cultural groups.
- Understand the consequences of lack of SC preparedness for MHDs.
- Become aware of the impact of community engagement during MHDs.
- Understand the strategic importance of equality, diversity, and inclusion (EDI) in the delivery of SC.
- Become aware about the possible contribution that can be made by technology during MHDs.
- Understand the need for training how to provide SC to multicultural patients during MHDs.
- Familiarize yourself with the need of a national strategy for providing SC during MHDs.

Introduction

None of us had experienced anything like the COVID pandemic before. It was "apocalyptic," a "war zone," a "hell," absolute "mayhem."

Papadopoulos et al., 2021

This chapter is based on a study undertaken by the author and colleagues in 2021 during the second peak of the COVID-19 pandemic in the United Kingdom. Its aim was to identify the components of a national strategy for the provision of SC to patients, their families, and staff during MHDs and emergencies. During MHDs, the demand for SC grows exponentially. Senior nurses and spiritual leaders alike bear a great responsibility for the patients' spiritual well-being and are an indispensable workforce during health emergencies. The study explored National Health Service (NHS) nurse managers' and NHS senior chaplains' experiences and views in relation to SC in England during the COVID-19 pandemic, from March 2020 to July 2021.

We interviewed 25 individuals, comprising 9 senior nurses and 16 senior chaplains. Among the latter, there were nine full-time NHS chaplains, all occupying senior roles, and the remainder were a mix of part-time and/or volunteer hospital chaplains with many years of experience, who often also were community faith representatives and/or working in independent social and healthcare organizations. Of the nursing managers included, four worked in critical care/EoL (end of life), whereas the other five were senior nurses working in other hospital areas. Over 50% of our participants had more than 16 years of experience in their job positions at the time of interview. The majority of participants worked in London (32%), others were based across six regions of England, and one was in the Isle of Man.

The first topic of the interview was: "Have you ever experienced a national health emergency like the COVID-19 pandemic during your career?"

Their replies are summarized as follows:

None of us had experienced anything like the COVID pandemic before. It was 'apocalyptic', a 'war zone', a 'hell', absolute 'mayhem'. During the first wave we were all scared. We were not prepared for such apocalyptic series of events. None of us knew how best to deal with this disease. The uncertainty and the unknowns exacerbated our anxiety. It was mayhem! We wanted to protect ourselves and we also worried in case we took the virus home to our families. Some of us decided to live in accommodation provided by our employers rather than risk infecting our families. Colleagues were really struggling both physically and mentally. We tried to support each other. The available hospital chaplains provided much needed spiritual support. They listened and they prayed for us and our families (summary from interviews of senior nurses).

Papadopoulos et al., 2021

Before I go any further, let me provide two relevant definitions that resulted from the findings of this study and one that did not. According to the study's participants, "*Spirituality is an integral part of all human beings which is connected to religions, faiths, personal philosophies, a relationship with ourselves, others and the environment, as well as a relationship with a transcendent superior force, which helps us understand the meaning and purpose of our existence and that of others.*"

SC in this study is described as an "*integral component of culturally competent and compassionate care*" (Papadopoulos, 2018). In this sense, SC indicates a broad and comprehensive spiritual presence, comfort, and other actions not only to patients but also to their loved ones as well as health workers. SC stems from an "*understanding [of] the suffering of others and wanting to do something about it [and] takes into consideration the patients' and the carers' cultural backgrounds as well as the context in which care is given*" (Papadopoulos, 2018, p. 2).

Koenig and Schultz (2016) defined an MHD as an event that causes serious disruption to the health and healthcare functions of a community. It involves extensive casualties and destruction and exceeds the response capacity of the affected area.

Natural and human-made disasters are dramatically increasing. According to the United Nations, cataclysmic events worldwide have tripled in the last 50 years (UN News, 2021). Within all types of disasters, MHDs are also on the rise worldwide (International Federation of Red Cross and Red Crescent Societies, 2018), and these have tremendous impacts on public health and the health systems of affected populations (Noji, 2000; Shoaf &

Rottman, 2000). The COVID-19 pandemic was an extreme, unprecedented existential global crisis, during which radical changes occurred in the provision of SC to hospitalized patients and their relatives. In particular, studies indicate that SC drastically diminished, due to the emergency burden of care of frontline healthcare workers, and the infection control precautions hampered the services of SC units in hospitals (Cockell, 2020; Papadopoulos et al., 2021). Although this was initially suggested, it is now evidenced that the outbreak caught healthcare providers and governments unprepared in terms of a national strategy for the provision of SC in MHDs.

The UN defined major disaster as a serious disruption of the functioning of a community or a society, involving widespread human, material, economic, or environmental losses and impacts, which exceeds the ability of the affected community or society to cope using its own resources (UNISDR, 2009). Major disasters of any kind have a tremendous impact on public health and the health systems of affected populations.

Here is a list of MHDs from the beginning of the 20th century to now:

- 1918 Spanish flu pandemic—A deadly influenza pandemic that infected around 500 million people worldwide. Began in early 1918 and lasted until 1920. Caused over 50 million deaths globally.
- HIV/AIDS pandemic—First recognized in 1981 when cases of rare pneumonias and cancers were reported in gay men in Los Angeles. HIV spread globally over the next decades, killing over 36 million people worldwide so far.
- 2002–2004 SARS outbreak—Severe acute respiratory syndrome (SARS) originated in China in 2002, quickly spreading to over two dozen countries. Resulted in over 8000 cases and 774 deaths before being contained.
- 2009 H1N1 swine flu pandemic—A novel strain of influenza A virus that originated in Mexico and the United States in early 2009. Spread globally and is estimated to have caused over 200,000 deaths.
- 2014–2016 West Africa Ebola epidemic—Worst Ebola outbreak to date started in Guinea in 2014 before spreading to other West African countries. Over 28,000 cases and 11,000 deaths.
- 2020–present COVID-19 pandemic—Novel coronavirus SARS-CoV-2 emerged in Wuhan, China, in late 2019. Rapidly spread worldwide, resulting in over 652 million confirmed cases and over 6.6 million deaths so far.

Lessons From COVID-19

LESSON 1: PROTECT AND SUPPORT THE WORKFORCE IN CULTURALLY COMPETENT AND COMPASSIONATE WAYS, BEFORE, DURING, AND AFTER MAJOR HEALTH DISASTERS AND EMERGENCIES

As we can see from the aforementioned list, during two MHDs in the 20th century, 86 million people died. During the first two decades of the 21st century, 7,587,000 people have lost their lives in four MHDs. Of course, these figures do not account the deaths that happened as a result of natural and human-made disasters. In addition, millions of people who escaped death, including nurses, were left with long-term physical and mental health problems.

Deaths and Moral Injuries

In the study we mentioned earlier, a number of chaplains and many senior nurses we interviewed found the huge number of deaths as a shocking phenomenon in itself, which was further exacerbated by the fact that several patients were dying without their relatives around. The emptiness and "unusual silence in the hospital" (8NSERosie) were very disturbing for staff, as they felt the patients' "isolated journey" (8NSERosie) and had to cope with a widespread "injustice of dying alone" (5CNWKen). Raising awareness about the shocking reality of huge numbers of deaths and the impact on the working environment must be part of any preparedness training of all nursing staff. Discussing these topics and helping the nurses develop coping strategies will be a positive and compassionate act of supporting the workforce, who will be better prepared to face the *"apocalyptic", "war zone", "hell"* of an MHD.

Apart from the effects of the disease, many senior nurses reported that their staff were suffering from "moral injury." This has been defined by the psychiatrist Jonathan Shay in 2009 as the psychological distress that results from actions, or lack thereof, which violate one's moral or ethical code (Shay, 2014). The words of those interviewed are summarized as follows:

Shift after shift we were witnessing death all around us. We tried our best to stay with the dying persons, as we wanted to comfort them and ease their fear of death by holding their hand or reading a prayer, but too often this was not possible as we were overwhelmed by all the physical care other patients needed to stay alive. The patients' loved ones were not allowed to visit, which was very sad and upsetting to them, to the patients and to the staff. Occasionally, if the dying person was a colleague, we made an exception and allowed a visitor. However, when this happened we felt guilty as we knew that our actions were creating care inequalities. This moral dilemma, on top of many others, such as being part in the decision to shut someone's ventilator and discontinue treatment, has been referred to by some as 'moral injury'. We would carry such injuries with us for a very long time. We will need to be supported and helped to heal our long-term trauma, as many of us will not be able to do this alone.

The notion of moral injury has been raised by several participants in different ways. This notion was often accompanied by a reflection on the need for long-term support for staff and the public too, in terms of collective bereavement and remembrance. Looking to the future, many interviewees also connected moral injury to the need for better preparation and training for all healthcare staff to be able to appropriately deal, professionally and emotionally, with death. One of the interviewees stated:

If there is going to be anything that comes out in a strategy or protocol or a policy from the evidence you are collecting, that should be about the importance of having skills and knowledge and experience on the ground to provide what is needed. This has been most well highlighted in hospitals where nurses who aren't used to a lot of deaths were handling death a lot which was overwhelming to them. (10CSWCat)

It is obvious that the nursing workforce needs support and training to develop coping strategies that will protect them from moral injuries (Cockell & McSherry, 2012). Learning about the meaning of moral injuries and how to recognize the symptoms and the impact they may have on them, as well as about the support the organization provides to them, will help the nursing professionals prevent or lessen the negative effects. It is therefore a moral obligation of employers to create a culturally competent and compassionate working environment and to provide regular opportunities for staff to engage in self-care practices such as mindfulness, meditation, exercise, self-compassion, and so on, both before and after an MHD or emergency.

Lack of Preparedness for Major Health Disasters

One senior chaplain we interviewed during the study mentioned earlier described how during the early stages of the pandemic, realizing that the team had no guidelines and no experience with pandemics, he discussed with them the need to prepare a short paper as quickly as they could, describing what they should be doing, the practical actions they could take, what to expect from the NHS Trust (their employer), and why. They presented their paper to the Trust's management board, which integrated it in their developing policies. He went on to add: *"Preparation is most important. The Trusts who will prepare well will fare the bests"* (13CNWFin).

The lack of preparedness has been widely discussed during and after the catastrophic peaks of the COVID-19 pandemic. Lack of preparedness affected everyone: the general public, the patients, and the workforce. In particular, many nurses suffered from the disease, some died from it, and some were left with the long-term effects of the disease. Sadly, many have since left the profession.

A preparedness strategy about culturally competent SC should be developed and enacted at regular intervals to enable the staff to gain experience in order to be prepared when the next MHD or major emergency happens. A strategy must have a clear protocol, including information about who will initiate it, who will coordinate the practice of it, who will participate in the practice, what additional training and other resources (such as protective equipment) the staff need in order to effectively and safely operate in infectious or other hazardous environments, what records might need to be kept, and how to debrief and support the spiritual providers, managers, and NHS/multicultural and multifaith volunteer chaplains so that their experiences and views are taken into consideration and needed changes and improvements can be included in the strategy.

Preparedness: Culturally Competent and Compassionate Training

Ongoing training of the workforce is one of the best ways to prepare the staff for future MHDs and emergencies. Since most communities and care teams are multicultural, the need for culturally competent and compassionate training is of utmost importance. Having a good understanding of cultural diversity will empower nurses to provide culturally appropriate and sensitive care to their patients in the most demanding emergencies. Important elements of this training should be about ethical decision-making and how to respond to ethical dilemmas related to cultural differences. A good way to adopt the training is that of simulations and scenarios that mimic the physical conditions and ethical dilemmas they may encounter in a crisis, allowing them to practice culturally competent spiritual and other care as well as ethical decision-making.

Preparedness training in culturally competent psychological first aid techniques will better equip the nursing workforce to provide emotional support to patients, families, and each other during emergencies. These examples will enforce the workforce's resilience, enable them to better manage their stress, and prevent or reduce moral injury.

Culturally and Compassionately Competent Spiritual Care

One of the senior nurses we interviewed in the project referred to earlier defined spirituality as "*a journey of discovery of one's own spirituality, …*". She went on to say that "*during the pandemic nurses were reflecting about the sources of their strength during the extreme COVID situations*" (9NLFlo).

There was no doubt in the minds of the study's participants that the pandemic not only emphasized the importance of SC but also offered the opportunity to redefine it in more secular and transcendent terms rather than only religious terms. Another interviewee stated:

Spiritual care isn't just about religious care. It's about caring for the individual. And all that individual brings. Hopes, fears, joys. Whatever. …spiritual care is there for everybody. Because we're all spiritual beings. We're not robots. (3CSEEvi)

The integration of SC in all policies was also recommended. One interviewee expanded further:

I have tried to raise the profile of the need for an integration of spiritual care into policy because it tends to get left out, and side-lined, and people are a bit nervous of what it means […]. And then the practical way of delivering that, […] the resources available, what can be drawn upon, what teams look like, what they can offer, but it is this overall idea that spiritual care is an essential component and if anything, it feels to me, as if the pandemic has shown just that. (10CSWCat)

It is evident from the data we collected that healthcare workers, especially nurses, urgently need to be prepared to:

- Conduct culturally competent spiritual/religious assessment of the needs of patients, which should be recorded in the official patient records;
- Report the SC interventions given to patients in their records; and
- Be assured that SC should be integrated in all policies related to MHDs.

Patients' needs may include culturally specific rituals used to help them and their families cope with the extreme trauma situations. It is wise to have the training include information about the rituals based on the cultural groups that live in specific communities. It is also important to develop accessible resources about the rituals of other cultural groups. During MHDs and emergencies, the priority is to save lives and to deal with the dying or dead individuals in culturally competent and compassionate ways. Here are some examples of rituals relating to dying, death, bereavement, and remembrance. Note that individuals or families belonging to the groups included in these examples may not follow these rituals, so nurses must always check with the patients or the families of the deceased. The text provided here is culture generic to the groups referred in the examples, which can raise the nurses' awareness and either start a conversation or, in the absence of family, be used as part of efforts to treat the incapacitated patient or the deceased with dignity and respect.

Dying rituals: Christians carry out the ritual of anointing and communion. These holy sacraments are given by a priest to very sick and dying persons. Anointing involves the laying of hands on the head of the person and the application of holy oil from the priest finger to the forehead of the sick and dying person. During the peaks of the COVID-19 pandemic, dying patients could no longer have these rituals. When a priest was available and the family requested the ritual of anointing, the priest used an ear bud to apply the holy oil.

Muslims hold prayer sittings, usually led by an imam. During the pandemic, Muslim patients had prayers via digital prayer cubes or other AI assistants.

Buddhist rituals include chanting and prayer ceremonies to help ease the transition of the soul and bring comfort to the individual.

Hindus recite sacred texts and perform chanting of religious verses, mantras, and prayers from Hindu scriptures to provide spiritual support.

Jewish rituals for the dying include visiting the sick and reciting psalms.

Funerals, bereavement, and remembrance rituals: Traditional Chinese funerals may include an organized mourning procession, with mourners wearing black or white clothes and family members wearing mourning bands. Burning paper money, houses, and cars is common to ensure that the deceased has a comfortable afterlife.

African cultures engage in traditional singing and dancing to express their emotions and find strength in unity during funerals and bereavement.

Islamic traditions of mourning include the washing of the body after death by family members of the same gender. The deceased is then wrapped in a white shroud. Islam emphasizes the swift burial of the deceased, preferably within 24 hours. Delaying the burial is discouraged. This is followed by 3 days of mourning. Families may organize sessions where the entire Quran is recited for the benefit of the deceased. The completion of the Quran is considered a form of supplication for the departed soul.

Jewish rituals for the deceased require that the body is washed, purified, and dressed in a simple white burial garment. It is then watched over until the burial, which should happen within 24 hours after the death.

Many cultures perform ancestor veneration to honor and connect with their deceased ancestors. The usual practice is to light candles, offer food, and offer specific prayers for guidance from their ancestors.

It must be noted that during the peaks of the COVID-19 pandemic, most of the rituals described earlier could not be followed, but modified versions were used. Due to the many restrictions, dying individuals could not have their families and spiritual/faith/religious persons around them to pray, sing, or perform other rituals for them. However, families could relay messages or videos of the rituals they conducted at home via a nurse who played these to the patients on a tablet or a phone. Due to the huge numbers of dead people, the burials could not take place in the required times and in the traditional ways. Funerals, mourning, and bereavement rituals were performed online if the technology was available.

Policy Development

Developing clear, ethical, and culturally competent policies and guidelines that address key issues such as resource allocation, triage, discontinuation of treatment, switching off a ventilator, and visitor restrictions during emergencies will help nurses navigate the challenges of future disasters and emergencies, ultimately supporting their well-being.

Research and Evaluation

Nurses must be empowered by their employers to conduct or to be involved in multidisciplinary research and yearly evaluation of the effectiveness of preparedness strategies to ensure that necessary adjustments are made and their organizations respond to any shortcomings or recommendations reported in their findings. Being proactive in this way will provide the assurance healthcare workers need in order to continue working in safe and supportive environments.

LESSON 2: PROTECT AND SUPPORT THE PUBLIC AND PATIENTS IN CULTURALLY COMPETENT AND COMPASSIONATE WAYS BEFORE AND AFTER MAJOR HEALTH DISASTERS AND EMERGENCIES

The COVID-19 pandemic created unprecedented challenges for nurses as they worked to provide quality care while protecting themselves and their patients. During the peaks of COVID-19 infections, nurses had to adapt quickly to new policies, equipment, and procedures while facing immense workloads. Providing culturally competent and compassionate care was more critical than ever, though often more difficult.

Nurses encountered patients and families from diverse backgrounds, who had differing perspectives and approaches to health and illness. Effective cross-cultural communication was essential but hampered by the personal protective equipment (PPE) and isolation protocols. Nurses made extra efforts to connect with patients as individuals, especially when their family were not allowed to visit.

Compassionate care was strained by the trauma of the pandemic. Nurses had to balance infection control policies with human connection. Holding a patient's hand while wearing gloves or being the only person present when a patient passed— these moments required immense compassion.

Community Engagement

During the pandemic, nurses and spiritual leaders tried to enhance and strengthen their connection with the public as well as building partnerships with community organizations. These activities enabled them to disseminate information about the pandemic and explain the reasons of the enforced strict rules.

During the 16 months of our project (March 2020 to July 2021), we often heard interviewees describing their own experiences of the COVID-19 pandemic as strange and stressful. At the same time, many people spoke about how the pandemic acted as a catalyst in bringing people and communities together. Moreno (2018) states that communities have the power to activate internal resilient capacities to cope with and recover from natural disasters. It is reasonable to suggest that this statement can be applied to MHDs. Moreno's study highlighted that communities are not simply passive victims of disasters but are also active agents. According to her, the term "resilience" originates from the Latin word *"resilio"*, which means "to jump back". The concept of resilience was popularized by the Hyogo Framework for Action (HFA, 2005–2015) (ISDR, 2007), which emphasized the need and the ways to build resilient communities. Colten and colleagues (2008) describe resilient communities in the disaster context as those that have the following capacities: integrated emergency institutions and communications; formal disaster plans; trained first responders; multi-hazard event response exercises; a reserve of personnel, material, and financial resources; public education and information; and continuing long-term planning for recovery and vulnerability reduction.

The participants in our study did indeed emphasize their observation that the pandemic brought people together in terms of both the healthcare workforce community and their local communities. Many declared that COVID-19 changed people's perspective of life. Healthcare staff and members of the local communities expressed the need to join meetings, events, and services, as they wanted to be part of something larger and more spiritual. One of our interviewees stated:

Different communities had different spiritual needs which related to spaces for contemplation, places of wellbeing awareness, food, and ways through which their voices were heard. (13CNWFin)

Another added:

We empowered local communities to find their own ways of remembering those who died. (5CNWKen)

Some interviewees reported that resilient communities were created during the pandemic when the local authorities, the NHS, and the local communities worked together for the common good. Engaging with communities provided opportunities, primarily to the chaplains, to work with and empower people and their locality.

The need to develop better working relationships with local communities was recognized by the participants of this study. The efforts made by the nurse leaders and chaplains to engage with their communities and to encourage dialogue enabled the voices of both health staff and the public to be heard, which resulted in a better understanding of what was going on and mutual appreciation of their realities. This was an example of victims being also active agents. The benefits of this proactive and compassionate SC manifested in the form of flexibility and willingness to accept the stringent changes in policy and practice. For example, relatives and patients came to accept the provision of SC by chaplains of any faith, by nurses, and by other healthcare staff.

Trust

Trust is the glue of life. It is the most essential ingredient in effective communication. It is the foundational principle that holds all relationships (Covey, 2004). Trust is closely connected to confidence, consistency, and communication. The data collected in our study spoke to the "surreal" COVID-19 pandemic time of uncertainty, confusion, high risk, and despair.

The nurse leaders reported that in the early stages of the pandemic, there were no specific protocols to follow in order to care for the COVID-19 patients and that the staff were doing the best they could using the available resources.

Government guidelines for hospitals and the public were constantly changing, sometimes contradicting previous advice, sometimes the guidelines were inconsistent across the United Kingdom, and at other times they seemed irrational and unfair. Participants stated that this lack of consistency, the volume of information being given on a daily basis, and the quality of information resulted in the loss of trust by many members of the public and to some extent by the healthcare staff. One of the senior nurses stated:

It is easy to lose trust, but hard to get it back. We had to work hard to win staff and public confidence and trust. (6NLJess)

Most of the participants included examples of how they tried to regain people's trust such as walking in the hospital grounds, talking to staff and family members, reassuring them, giving them information, and listening to them. Hospital Trusts realized that to gain the staff's trust and confidence, they should take actions that assured their safety and responded to their psychological and spiritual needs. A number of initiatives were put in place some weeks into the first peak of the pandemic. Some chaplains went even further as they reached out and engaged with their communities, providing compassion circles, intergenerational and age-related online sharing groups, and other opportunities for spiritual support. All these activities helped people remain positive and informed. Disseminating useful information

and reliable and compassionate messages was also reported by some chaplains who took part in radio programs and discussions.

Clear Communication

In extreme, urgent, and complex healthcare situations, effective communication becomes absolutely essential. It helps us connect with one another, share values, knowledge, and experiences, support others, and grieve and rejoice with others, and it is the main tool for the giving and receiving SC.

As the various multidisciplinary and often multicultural and multifaith teams were trying to prepare the services needed, to deliver these under chaotic and fast-changing conditions, and to review their practices and results, cross-team communication was paramount as well as challenging. During the COVID-19 pandemic, many levels of communication were in operation: between members of frontline clinical staff, between caregivers and patients, caregivers, and families of patients, between clinical and nonclinical staff, between management and service givers, between management and NHS departments, and so on.

Communication is not just verbal; the vast proportion of communication is nonverbal, through facial expressions, gestures—the ultimate gesture being that of a smile (Axtell, 2008)—tone and volume of voice, positions and distance of the persons trying to communicate (often referred to as proxemics), all of which are molded by everyone's own culture, which means that gestures can both enhance and inhibit communication.

Participants of this study reported barriers and enablers to communication, such as the challenges they experienced trying to communicate while in full PPE:

In terms of the barrier that PPE causes, I remember early on I said to a patient—I'm sorry I've got this mask on. You can't see I'm smiling, and she said, I can see you're smiling from your eyes. So, although clearly, for lip reading there are issues, but in terms of being able to make human connection that is still possible. I had trouble with goggles steaming up so I'm reading prayers and peering through the edge of the goggle to try and see the words I'm trying to read off the page … it was hard to communicate through PPE, but we found ways out of this…. (6CEMJon)

One of the chaplains we interviewed referred to the importance of having short conversations with staff and placing simple items in the hospital chapel to show that hope and love comprise a powerful message. He said:

Some of our most poignant conversations have been with the cleaners and the security guards, because they have to be very present, they are aware of what's going on. We have some lovely interactions with them, we're all human, and what's going on around us affects everybody, and I think this particular pandemic, there's no boundaries between what's happening in hospital and what's happening at homes. So, we put some stones in the chapel with some words on them like 'love', 'hope', and 'peace', and one of the security guards came in and said he'd like to take one for his daughter, …and he was going to give it to his daughter and just to tell her that he was going to be ok, and if she was worried about him to maybe hold the stone, say a little prayer for him, and little things like that. And it was quite an eye-opener as to how much people observed, and carried the burden as a whole organisation, really. (4CNWNick)

LESSON 3: EQUALITY, DIVERSITY, AND INCLUSION

The issue of EDI was raised by several interviewees. One of the specific topics frequently discussed revolved around volunteer chaplains and minority faiths. The fact that in almost all Trusts volunteer chaplains were not allowed to visit the hospitals meant that many patients following minority faiths and wanting specific cultural–religious support could not receive it. In fact, the NHS employed chaplains in most hospitals who belong to a few religions, chiefly Christianity and its different branches. However, religious support needs, including specific rites, span across the great variety of religions present in England, and catering to such a rich variety of religious needs is essentially in the hands of community faiths leaders volunteering in hospitals and of part-time NHS chaplains. Despite the fact that SC has universal application, visiting restrictions during the pandemic meant that patients and families from minority faiths were more deprived in terms of receiving support for their specific religious and SC needs, given in a culturally competent way by their community faith leaders.

One of our interviewees stated:

Religious care for minority faiths during COVID was disabled. Volunteers' access to hospital was taken away, and volunteer chaplains were only occasionally called by an NHS chaplain to take care of minority faiths' patients. (1CLBob)

Another said:

There are questions about human rights, and for some people access to religious care would be seen as a human right. Families might be very distressed that somebody who really would have wanted prayer and support at the end of life hasn't had it. (5CNWKen)

Others had more positive statements:

We're fortunate that we have a good team in that we have other chaplains, bank chaplains, who are from different religious traditions. (2CEMAda)

When one specific chaplain from a specific faith was missing and was requested by a patient, we managed to have someone from that faith come in. (13CNWFin)

The issue of EDI was also linked to hospital visiting policies. Several participants pointed out the need for more compassionate rules, within, of course, the boundaries of safety and protection for all. Such a policy would be beneficial, as an occasional visit by a member of the family would provide relief to both patients and family. Staff would also benefit spiritually, as the knowledge that dying patients were able to see a loved one would lessen their sadness and spiritual pain. A senior nurse leader reported that the very strict visiting policy aroused a sense of injustice in her and some other staff, which led them to occasionally break the government regulations, which, in turn, led to moral injuries because not all patients were having the same benefit.

One interviewee described the visiting policy:

We were quite regularly reviewing the visiting policy to assess whether we were doing the right thing, telling families not to come in, and whether we needed to make exceptions, and how did that. It's quite a chaotic way of working. I'm not sure it is sustainable. I also do worry that there was some inequality in the decisions we made around which visitors could come in and who couldn't. We went the extra mile when it was a member of staff who was dying, and I understand why, but we did more for that person than we did for other people, and I'm not sure how we justify that. You know, I think that's not, right. (4CNWNick)

It is clearly evident that in order to implement equitable and inclusive visiting policies, it is necessary to have resources to do that safely. For this, PPE and other resources become indispensable. Furthermore, like the policies, infection control resources should be inclusive and culturally competent too.

LESSON 4: TECHNOLOGY

The use of information and communication technologies (ICTs) proved to be central in several realms of people's lives during the COVID-19 pandemic, and SC was no exception. Relatives who could not visit their loved ones in hospitals, chaplains who were shielding and could be neither in the wards nor in their hospital offices, and spiritual leaders whose places of worships had to be closed had to rely on ICTs in order to provide and receive SC. Almost all interviewees reported that physical presence and SC were much more effective than the virtual option, which often was the only one. However, several participants also highlighted how using ICTs allowed shielding chaplains to continue their role from home. For this, they lamented how virtual connections were initially hampered by the lack of devices.

We were fortunate that we were given tablets and smartphones as well. I know that my colleagues who were shielding were able to use those to provide support for patients and families and found that really helpful, because it meant that they felt able to be part of things. (2CEMAda)

We did also find there was a problem and a delay in accessing some ICT equipment, due to global demand at the beginning of the pandemic. So even if we wanted to get more tablets into homes to make this kind of connection, it was difficult. (11CEM+Norb)

We used ICTs on the wards, where the families couldn't attend, and on the whole my experience was quite positive … I've had nurses holding a tablet with the family able to be present via their tablet, and I was able to share a prayer or blessing at the bedside. (4CNWNick)

A very important … and helpful [thing] during the pandemic, apart from going in [to the hospital] ourselves, has been remote connectivity. Especially as minority faiths, rather than having to travel long distances, it is just enough to connect, even if you are far away from the hospital, there is no travel delay, and they are secure connections and they give us the ability to intervene wherever we are requested. (1CLBob)

ICTs also allowed the conduction of rituals—mostly funerals, or other EoL rites—for patients and their families despite these having to be modified sometimes. Important memorial services and other virtual gatherings could only happen thanks to ICTs, and in fact, some participants underlined how they could do things never done before thanks to ICTs.

Thinking about the difficulty that some categories of people, as well as EoL patients, could experience in using devices that entail touch, reading, and memory, in the context of highly contagious environment, intelligent, autonomous, and mobile robots could really help reduce contamination spreading.

An interviewee stated:

What has worked really well, I think, they're called portals, and the thing about portals is that it's just end-to-end. So, you have an icon, you press it and it just pings on your son's tablet, so instead of having to go into Zoom, get the right thing. So, I think those and voice-operated artificially intelligent (AI) systems such as perhaps an AI assistant [the name of the device], where if the person has mental capacity and they're able to say "… [the name of the device], can you phone my granddaughter," or a surgery or whatever else it is. So, I think technology offers a lot. (11CEM+Norb)

Our findings about using technology to provide spiritual support to patients are summarized as follows:

As chaplains and nurses, we realised early on that in order to reach our patients and their families we had to be creative, inventive and, for the first time in some cases, started using known but not practising ways of communicating and providing support. We began to use computer tablets, mobile phones (sometimes our own), to connect patients with their loved ones to give and receive spiritual support. Many times, we had to read messages from family members to the patients, and vice versa, as patients were too weak and breathless to do so themselves. We also streamed religious/faith services to patients and the community. In the early stages of the pandemic, we struggled with the technology as we tried to do things we never did before. We also did not have the number of technological devices we needed. But we are sure that without them, all of us would have been more isolated and would have far fewer opportunities to give and receive the much needed spiritual support that nourished our souls during this unprecedented existential crisis.

LESSON 5: VACCINATION HESITANCY

The IENE 11 PROVAC project—*"Empowering nurses and healthcare professionals to promote vaccination and tackle vaccine hesitancy"* (https://ieneproject.eu/IENE11/about-project.php)—conducted by my colleagues, addressed the issue of vaccination hesitancy during the pandemic and beyond. This project aimed to support and train the healthcare professionals to address vaccine hesitancy in a culturally competent way, to improve vaccine confidence, to enhance their knowledge on vaccination, to tackle the misinformation and disinformation, and to ensure clear communication on the benefits, risks, and importance of COVID-19 vaccines.

Vaccinations are one of the most significant achievements in the history of medicine, playing a pivotal role in preventing and controlling the spread of infectious diseases. As the world grappled with the COVID-19 pandemic, the importance of vaccinations became more pronounced than ever.

During the COVID-19 pandemic, vaccination rates were found to be lower among people belonging to ethnic minority populations and other underserved and socioeconomically disadvantaged groups. In addition, misinformation about the COVID-19 vaccination was spread through the social media, creating an urgency for health campaigns to provide factual, culturally and linguistically appropriate messaging (Gaughan et al., 2022).

As the world confronts the challenges posed by the COVID-19 pandemic, the urgency of culturally competent vaccination efforts cannot be overstated. Through the widespread adoption of COVID-19 vaccines, we have a powerful means to curb the spread of the virus, protect individuals from severe illness, and pave the way for a global recovery. Embracing vaccinations is not merely a personal choice; it is a collective responsibility to safeguard public health and build a resilient global community; however, this can be achieved only if information and messages provided are inclusive, in the various languages, sensitively acknowledging the concerns by educating the diverse communities and their leaders, and by providing easily accessible vaccination centres.

The IENE 11 PROVAC project contributed in the aforementioned efforts through the following activities:

- By developing a database of reliable sources of information and tools on different issues on vaccines and vaccination. (Download the Information Guide on Vaccination & Vaccination Hesitancy.)
- By developing a set of 20 information sheets presenting the essential, reliable, and evidence-based information on various vaccine and vaccination issues with the aim of combating misinformation and fake news, debunking myths, and discouraging the vaccine hesitancy, available in English, Romanian, Greek, and Spanish (EN, RO, EL, and ES).
- By developing a culturally competent training curriculum in EN, RO, EL, and ES.

- By developing 20 bite-sized learning tools also available in EN, RO, EL, and ES.
- By delivering a Massive Open Online Course (MOOC).

(All outputs can be freely downloaded at https://ieneproject.eu/IENE11/about-project.php and https://iene11.eu/.)

The pandemic magnified preexisting healthcare disparities and barriers across populations. Learning from the lessons I have discussed in this chapter will promote progress through giving diverse communities greater voice alongside nurses and leaders in codesigning systemic reforms that better meet the needs of our increasingly pluralistic societies. Cultural competence must move beyond awareness toward action.

Posthumanism, COVID-19, and Major Disasters

The progress we expect to make following the COVID-19 pandemic will be more positive if we include elements of new theories such as the posthumanist theory. As stated in previous chapters, the posthuman theory explores the ways in which technology, particularly biotechnology and artificial intelligence, is challenging and redefining traditional notions of what it means to be human. It considers how emerging technologies could potentially alter human biology, cognition, and consciousness.

While the direct application of posthuman theory to specific health disasters may not be straightforward, it provides a framework for critical analysis and reflection on the ways in which technology intersects with human experiences, societal structures, and ethical considerations during times of crisis. As future health disasters unfold, the posthuman perspective may become increasingly relevant in shaping discussions on the role of technology in responding to and mitigating the impact of such events.

Posthumanist discussions often revolve around the ethical implications of emerging technologies. One such ethical implication that was identified by the study we referred to earlier was about the inequalities regarding access to technology. Posthuman theory encourages reflection on how emerging technologies may exacerbate or alleviate social and economic disparities during major disasters, including major health emergencies.

An example of biotechnological interventions is that of vaccination technology. The rapid development of vaccines for COVID-19 showcases the role of biotechnology in addressing health crises. This aligns with posthumanist ideas where technology is not just a tool but an integral part of human evolution.

The pandemic has also accelerated the adoption of digital health solutions, including telemedicine. From a posthumanist standpoint, these technologies blur the lines between the physical and digital realms and traditional notions of healthcare delivery.

Summary and Recommendations

This chapter's primary focus was to present some of the culture-generic and culture-specific SC challenges that the UK nursing workforce faced during the first 3 years of the COVID-19 pandemic and to reflect on the lessons we learned and those we will be learning in the near future.

To begin with, the key definitions such as MHDs, spirituality, and SC were given, followed up by a summary table of MHDs during the 20th and 21st centuries. This provided at a glance the extent of the global devastation and loss of life. More than 95 million people lost their lives during the MHDs listed in the 20th and 21st centuries so far.

Drawing on the findings of a study conducted in 2020–2021 (Papadopoulos et al., 2021) in the United Kingdom, we learned the importance of effective and compassionate leadership in order to protect and support the nursing workforce before, during, and after an MHD such as the COVID-19 pandemic. Nurses reported that they had never before encountered the size and ferocity of an MHD, and at the early stages of the pandemic they felt unprepared and unsupported. Protecting themselves and their families was an issue that created huge anxieties, particularly because colleagues became victims of the disease, which meant a lot of suffering and, in some cases, death. The volume of deaths among the patients was overwhelming, imposing exhausting workloads in depressing workplaces. Nurses also reported moral injuries due to the ethical decisions they had to make or be involved in, such as the dilemma of providing SC to the dying or providing care to save a patient, do they ignore the government guidelines (such as the prohibition of visitors) or do they stick to them, do they agree with the decision of the healthcare team to remove life support or do they dare to disagree, and so on. Nurses were physically, psychologically, and morally impacted, and we now know that a number of them will continue to suffer for a long time.

Engaging with the public proved to be a positive strategy, as nurses and chaplains working in hospitals and the community were able to provide information and support, which resulted in acts of compassion toward the more vulnerable community members. Study participants reported that communities became more resilient and hopeful. Participants credited the successful community engagement to the available technology, which allowed them to bring communities together and offer hope and opportunities to simply listen to the people's voices and demonstrate that they were all in this crisis together, even though they could not physically be together.

During the pandemic, inequalities were identified, particularly those affecting minority groups. These have been reported in the Public Health England 2020 report, "*Disparities in the risk and outcomes of COVID-19*". The highest age standardized diagnosis rates of COVID-19 per 100,000 population were in people of Black ethnic groups (486 in females and 649 in males) and the lowest were in people of White ethnic groups (220 in females and 224 in males). An analysis of survival among confirmed COVID-19 cases shows that, after accounting for sex, age, deprivation, and region, people of Bangladeshi ethnicity had around twice the risk of death when compared to people of White British ethnicity. People of Chinese, Indian, Pakistani, Other Asian, Black Caribbean, and Other Black ethnicity had between 10% and 50% higher risk of death when compared to White British ethnicity. Death rates from COVID-19 were higher for Black and Asian ethnic groups when compared to White ethnic groups. These disparities require urgent attention in order to achieve the goals of EDI.

This brief summary underlines the importance of supporting and training nursing staff in dealing with the multiple issues created during an MHD. It is imperative that staff well-being is taken care of, to ensure they can continue to provide high-quality, culturally competent SC. To achieve this, a clear and comprehensive strategy must be developed at the national level, which should be reviewed and enacted every year.

Activity

- Open or download the report "*Towards a national strategy for the provision of spiritual care and support during major health disasters*" by clicking the following link: https://cultureandcompassion.com/spirituality
- Once there, choose 'report 2'. If you have time, read the whole report (75 pages).
- Select one of the 11 components we recommended for a national strategy for the provision of SC and support during MHDs (pages 56–60), and write a short essay of 1000 words from any perspective you wish.
- Share with your work colleagues or fellow students.
- I recommend that you also try to publish your essay, either internally or in a national magazine/journal.

REFERENCES

Axtell, R. E. (2008). *Gestures: The do's and taboos of body language around the world*. 1st edition. Wiley.

Cockell, N. (2020). COVID-19 and grief: A chaplain's reflection on the experience of supporting bereaved parents and widows in lockdown. *Health and Social Care Chaplaincy, 8*.

Cockell, N., & McSherry, W. (2012). Spiritual care in nursing: an overview of published international research. *Journal of Nursing Management, 20*, 958–969. https://doi.org/10.1111/j.1365-2834.2012.01450.x.

Colten, C. E., Kates, R. W., & Laska, S. B. (2008). Community resilience:Lessons from New Orleans and hurricane Katrina, CARRI Report 3. Community and regional resilience initiative. chrome- extension://efaidnbmnnnibpcajpcglclefindmkaj/https://biotech.law.lsu.edu/climate/docs/a2008.03.pdf.

Covey, S. R. (2004). *The 7 habits of highly effective people: Powerful lessons in personal change, revisited edition*. Free Press.

Gaughan, C. H., et al. (2022). COVID-19 vaccination uptake amongst ethnic minority communities in England: a linked study exploring the drivers of differential vaccination rates. *Journal of Public Health, 44*. 4 (936). https://doi.org/10.1093/pubmed/fdac021.

International Federation of Red Cross, Red Crescent Societies. (2018). *World disasters report 2018: Leaving no one behind*. International Federation of Red Cross and Red Crescent Societies. https://www.ifrc.org/document/world-disasters-report-2018.

ISDR, (2007). Hyogo Framework for Action 2005-2015; Building the resilience of nations and communities to disasters. United Nations International Strategy for Disaster Reduction. Geneva, Switzerland.

Koenig, K. L., & Schultz, C. H. (Eds.). (2016). *Koenig and Schultz's disaster medicine comprehensive principles and practice* (2nd ed.). Cambridge University Press.

Moreno, J. (2018). The role of communities in coping with natural disasters: Lessons from the 2010 Chile Earthquake and Tsunami. Procedia Engineering, 7th International Conference on Building Resilience; Using scientific knowledge to inform policy and practice in disaster risk reduction 212, 1045. https://doi.org/10.1016/j.proeng.2018.01.134.

Noji, E. K. (2000). The public health consequences of disasters: Prehospital and disaster. *Medicine, 15*, 21–31. https://doi.org/10.1017/S1049023X00025255.

Papadopoulos, I. (2018). *Culturally competent compassion*. Routledge.

Papadopoulos, I., Lazzarino, R., Wright, S., Ellis Logan, P., & Koulouglioti, C. (2021). Spiritual support during COVID-19 in England: A scoping study of online sources. *J Relig Health, 60*, 2209–2230. https://doi.org/10.1007/s10943-021-01254-1.

Papadopoulos, I., Lazzarino, R., Koulouglioti, C., Ali, S., & Wright, S. (2021). *Towards a National Strategy for the Provision of Spiritual Care and Support in Major Health Disasters*. https://doi.org/10.13140/RG.2.2.15753.57445.

Shay, J. (2014). Moral injury. *Psychoanalytic Psychology, 31*(2), 182–191. doi:10.1037/a0036090.

Shoaf, K., & Rottman, S.J. (2000). Public health impact of disasters. *Australian Journal of Emergency Management, 15*, 58–63.

UNISDR. (2009). UNISDR terminology on disaster risk reduction.

UN News. (2021). *Natural disasters occurring three times more often than 50 years ago: new FAO report*. UN News. URL https://news.un.org/en/story/2021/03/1087702.

Chapter 6

Cultural Competence in AI and Robotics: Implications for Healthcare and Nursing

Learning Objectives

After reading this chapter, you should:

- Enhance your knowledge about cultural competence in healthcare and the evolution of artificial intelligence (AI) robotics.
- Become aware about the latest AI revolutionary language models (LMs).
- Appreciate the needs for ethics in the era of AI innovations and robots.
- Discover the importance of listening to the voices of patients and health professionals when designing and evaluating AI and robotics innovations.
- Reflect on posthuman perspectives of AI and robotics.

Introduction

This chapter begins with a brief exploration of the importance of cultural competence, the evolution of AI robotics, and how these two entities can intersect. The second section investigates the latest AI innovations such as the language models (LMs), for example ChatGPT. The use of LMs in healthcare and how these can promote cultural competence in healthcare and nursing are suggested. The third section discusses the fastest-growing subfield of AI, which is ethics, and provides an example of how ethics were applied in the *CARESSES* project. The fourth section highlights the importance of the involvement of diverse patient populations and healthcare workers, as early as possible, for researching and designing AI systems and of course during pilot projects. The last section discusses connections of posthuman perspectives of AI and culturally competent robots. Although currently most AI and robots lack cultural competency—the ability to understand and interact appropriately with different human cultures—as we learned in Chapter 2, posthumanists argue that we need to recognize the agency and importance of nonhuman entities in shaping human culture and society. It is inevitable that advance technology will continue to develop and be embedded in all health and social care institutions. The benefits are gradually being recognized, but there remain many challenges, such as responding to the lack of culturally competent robots and AI devices in both language and other forms of human communication.

Cultural Competence in Healthcare and the Evolution of AI Robotics

I declared my enthusiasm for technology at the very beginning of this book. So, let me add some more information about AI and robotics technologies in this chapter.

In 2023, three AI influential individuals provided the following views (https://kiboshib.com/5-powerful-quotes-about-ai-from-famous-people-2023/):

"These tools [AI] will help us to be more productive (can't wait to spend less time doing email!), healthier (AI medical advisors for people who can't afford care), smarter (students using ChatGPT to learn), and more entertained (AI memes lolol)," declared Sam Altman, CEO of OpenAI.

On the other hand, Elon Musk, CEO of X (former Twitter), Tesla, and SpaceX, made this statement: *"Mark my words…AI (artificial intelligence), is far more dangerous than the nukes."*

Sundar Pichai, CEO of Google's Alphabet, espoused that *"artificial intelligence will have a more profound impact in humanity than fire, electricity and the Internet."*

These are three interesting quotes from some of the pioneers of AI. Although not directly relevant to the topic of this chapter, they nevertheless address fundamental views we need to be aware of as we embrace more and more AI and robotics in nursing and the wider landscape of healthcare. For example, Altman refers to the impact of AI on health and education, two of the fields nurses and healthcare professionals can contribute to and/or apply in their work. Pichai emphasizes the colossal positive impact of AI that is advancing at a fast pace. Musk warns us of possible AI catastrophes that may occur if we are not careful, wise, and ethical in the development and usage of AI technologies.

Let me now remind us that cultural competence in healthcare refers to the ability of healthcare professionals and systems to provide care that respects and considers the cultural beliefs, values, practices, and needs of diverse patient populations. It is a critical aspect of providing effective and equitable healthcare, acknowledging the unique backgrounds and perspectives of individuals. As technology continues to transform the healthcare landscape, the integration of AI and robotics introduces new dimensions to the delivery of care.

DEFINITION AND IMPORTANCE OF CULTURAL COMPETENCE IN HEALTHCARE

As discussed in Chapter 2, cultural competence in healthcare is grounded in the understanding that individuals from different cultural backgrounds may have unique health beliefs, behaviors, and needs. It also involves the ability to effectively communicate, collaborate, and provide care to patients from diverse cultures, ensuring that their cultural, social, and linguistic factors are considered. The importance of cultural competence in healthcare is multifaceted, as we discovered in the previous chapters of this book.

But let me remind us of some of the benefits of culturally competent care. First, it enhances patient–provider communication. Effective communication is fundamental to quality healthcare, and when providers are culturally competent, they can bridge language and cultural gaps, leading to better understanding and trust between the healthcare professional and the patient.

Second, cultural competence contributes to better health outcomes. Patients are more likely to adhere to treatment plans and engage in preventive care when their cultural perspectives are acknowledged and integrated into their healthcare experience. This, in turn, can lead to improved overall health and well-being among diverse populations.

Third, cultural competence is crucial for reducing health inequalities. Many minority groups face inequalities in healthcare access, which impacts their health outcomes. Cultural competence helps address these inequalities by ensuring that healthcare services are tailored to the specific needs of different cultural groups, thereby promoting health equity.

EVOLUTION OF AI AND ROBOTICS IN HEALTHCARE

In 1955, the scientist John McCarthy and his colleagues (McCarthy et al., 1955) coined the term *artificial intelligence*, or *AI*, to describe the science and engineering of making intelligent machines. The evolution of AI robotics in healthcare represents a significant leap forward in the quest for more efficient, accurate, and accessible nursing and medical services, all of which are gradually becoming culturally competent too. Initially, AI in healthcare focused on improving diagnostic capabilities and treatment planning. For example, AI enabled the development of devises that can analyze medical images and identify patterns indicative of various conditions. This has not only increased the speed and accuracy of diagnostics but also allowed for more culturally appropriate personalized treatment plans.

The origins of medical AI robotics can be traced back to the mid-1980s when the PUMA 560 robotic surgical arm was used in neurosurgical biopsies (Kwoh et al., 1988). Since then, AI robotics have become commonplace in surgeries. The da Vinci system, approved in 2000, introduced robotic surgery assisted by AI with high-definition 3D vision (Lanfranco et al., 2004). Robotic surgery has expanded across specialties including urology, gynecology, and cardiology, allowing for minimally invasive procedures with greater precision.

Beyond surgical applications, AI robotics have been incorporated into rehabilitation practices. Myomo robotic is a myoelectric—the term refers to electric impulses generated by muscles of the body—AI robotic arm that enables a person with a weak or partially paralyzed arm to perform activities of daily living, such as feeding, reaching, and lifting. Socially assistive robots, for example the interactive therapeutic seal Paro, are able to stimulate the cognitive functions of people with dementia or Alzheimer disease that result in an emotional expression and response. This type of robots that are being used in nursing homes and research has found that they provide the user comfort and a sense of safety (Moyle et al., 2019). The *CARESSES* (Culturally Aware Robots and Environmental Sensor Systems for Elderly Support) project (2017–2021), a European Union (EU)–Japanese collaboration, created the first experimental, culturally competent assistive humanoid robot that can adapt the way it behaves and speaks to the culture of the person it is assisting (Papadopoulos & Koulouglioti, 2022).

Telemedicine, facilitated by AI, has expanded access to healthcare services, particularly in remote or underserved areas. Virtual consultations, remote monitoring, and AI-driven chatbots contribute to more accessible and timely healthcare, breaking down geographical barriers.

THE INTERSECTION OF CULTURAL COMPETENCE AND AI ROBOTICS

As AI robotics becomes more prevalent in healthcare, it is imperative to explore how these technological advancements intersect with the standards of cultural competence. While there may not be universally agreed-upon standards for cultural competence, many organizations and scholars have outlined key principles that contribute to cultural competence. In the United States, the widely recognized National Standards for Culturally and Linguistically Appropriate Services (CLAS) in Health and Health Care, developed by the Office of Minority Health, which is a part of the US Department of Health and Human Services, is used. The National CLAS Standards were first developed in 2000 and were reviewed and enhanced in 2013 (Office of Minority Health, 2013).

The enhanced CLAS standards are intended as guidelines and recommendations, not as legal mandates. However, the CLAS guidelines have informed laws, regulatory standards, and accreditation requirements aimed at promoting health equity and cultural/linguistic competency in healthcare. Adherence to the CLAS standards can help organizations meet broader legal and compliance requirements related to serving diverse patient populations.

The enhanced National CLAS Standards are structured as follows:
- Principal Standard (Standard 1): Provide effective, equitable, understandable, and respectful quality care and services that are responsive to diverse cultural health beliefs and practices, preferred languages, health literacy, and other communication needs
- Governance, Leadership, and Workforce (Standards 2–4)
- Communication and Language Assistance (Standards 5–8)
- Engagement, Continuous Improvement, and Accountability (Standards 9–15)

The integration of AI in healthcare has the potential to either reinforce or mitigate existing health inequalities based on cultural factors. One aspect of this intersection is the development of culturally sensitive AI algorithms. Recognizing that biases can exist in algorithms (as they also do in humans), efforts should be made to ensure that AI systems are trained on diverse datasets, avoiding reinforcement of existing healthcare inequalities. This involves incorporating cultural nuances into the algorithms to better understand and respond to the diverse needs of patient populations.

In terms of the principle of linguistic appropriate services, AI robots are well placed to speak many languages, thus limiting the inequalities created due to lack of communication and miscommunication. However, attention must be urgently given to issues such as variations in dialects, accents, and idioms. Furthermore, communication methods should adapt to patient disabilities such as those of hearing, vision, or cognition. Socially assistive robots also need sensitivities surrounding physical touch, personal space, eye contact, and privacy considerations, which vary across cultures.

It is important to mention that AI-driven chatbots and virtual assistants are able to provide patients with information, answer queries, and offer support in managing chronic conditions. All these examples correlate with the first and third CLAS standards, but we can easily discover intersection examples about the second and fourth principles of the enhanced CLAS standards.

AI robotics can play a role in boosting cultural competence among healthcare professionals. Virtual reality simulations and AI-driven training modules can immerse healthcare providers in scenarios that require culturally competent decision-making. This innovative approach helps build compassion, understanding, and effective communication skills, preparing providers to navigate diverse cultural contexts.

Despite these potential benefits, challenges exist at the intersection of cultural competence and AI robotics. Ensuring that AI systems are inclusive and culturally competent requires ongoing efforts to address biases in data, algorithms, and design. Additionally, the digital divide, where certain populations may have limited access to AI-driven healthcare technologies, must be considered in order to avoid exacerbating existing inequalities.

In summary, the intersection of cultural competence and AI robotics in healthcare represents a dynamic and evolving landscape. Cultural competence remains a cornerstone of providing equitable and effective healthcare, and as AI continues to reshape the healthcare ecosystem, it is essential to consider the cultural implications of these technological advancements. The integration of AI robotics has the potential to enhance cultural competence among healthcare professionals, improve patient outcomes, and contribute to the reduction of health disparities. However,

careful attention must be paid to address biases and ensure that these technologies are accessible to all, regardless of cultural background. As we navigate this intersection, it is crucial to approach the integration of AI in healthcare with a commitment to cultural competence, fostering a healthcare system that truly meets the diverse needs of its population.

The Latest AI Revolution With a Huge Future

The latest AI innovations are the LMs such as the ChatGPT. I asked one of them to explain what LMs are and to provide some examples of LMs as well as to suggest how these can promote cultural competence in healthcare and nursing. This is the answer I received:

LMs are AI systems that are trained on vast amounts of text data to learn patterns and relationships in language. They can then be used to generate human-like text, answer questions, summarize information, and assist with various language-related tasks.

Some existing LMs include the following:
1. GPT-3 (Generative Pre-trained Transformer 3) by OpenAI
2. BERT (Bidirectional Encoder Representations from Transformers) by Google
3. XLNet by Carnegie Mellon University and Google Brain
4. RoBERTa by Facebook AI Research
5. ALBERT (A Lite BERT) by Google Research and Toyota Technological Institute at Chicago

These LMs can promote cultural competence in healthcare and nursing in several ways:
1. Translation and interpretation: LMs can assist in translating medical information,

instructions, and communication between healthcare providers and patients who speak different languages, helping bridge language barriers and ensure understanding.

2. Cultural sensitivity in communication: By training LMs on diverse data sets that represent different cultural backgrounds, these models can help healthcare providers communicate in a more culturally sensitive manner, avoiding potential misunderstandings or offenses.

3. Patient education: LMs can help create patient education materials that are tailored to the cultural background and literacy level of patients, improving their understanding of health information and instructions.

4. Research and analysis: LMs can assist in analyzing large amounts of healthcare data to identify potential cultural biases or disparities in healthcare delivery, helping inform more culturally competent practices.

5. Personalized healthcare: By understanding a patient's cultural background and preferences, LMs can help healthcare providers tailor their approach and recommendations to the individual patient, promoting better patient engagement and adherence to treatment plans.

In summary, LMs can be a powerful tool for promoting cultural competence in healthcare and nursing by facilitating communication, education, research, and personalized care that recognizes and respects the diversity of patients' cultural backgrounds. However, it is important to note that while these LMs can be valuable tools, human involvement and oversight are crucial to ensure ethical use, prevent biases, and address the limitations of AI in understanding complex cultural contexts. Healthcare education and practice should thoughtfully adopt these models with a focus on enhancing, not replacing, human interaction and judgment.

Ethics in the Era of AI Innovations and Robots

Ethics are the fastest-growing subfield of AI, and almost all companies, governments, and nongovernmental international organizations involved in AI and robotics establish ethics teams to discuss the huge challenges faced by the sector. For example, the various UNESCO's reports (2018, 2019, 2020, 2021) on AI ethics stress the need for AI to be developed and deployed in ways that respect human dignity, democracy, justice, privacy, diversity, and sustainable development. Their work aims to provide ethical frameworks to harness AI's benefits while mitigating risks. According to Klaus Schwab (2016), the new era of AI and robotics is already changing how we live, work, and communicate. It is reshaping all aspects of government, such as education, healthcare, and commerce. It can change our relationships, our opportunities, our identities, and even, in some cases, our bodies as it changes the physical and virtual worlds we inhabit. It is already changing the things we value and the way we value them. This statement clearly raises a number of ethical challenges that need urgent attention.

One large company that has developed detailed principles and a code for ethical conduct is Google. In 2017, its DeepMind blog declared that they

...believe AI can be of extraordinary benefit to the world, but only if held to the highest ethical standards. Technology is not value neutral, and technologists must take responsibility for the ethical and social impact of their work. As history attests, technological innovation in itself is no guarantee of broader social progress. The development of AI creates important and complex questions. Its impact on society—and on all our lives—is not something that should be left to chance. Beneficial outcomes and protections against harms must be actively fought for and built-in from the beginning. But in a field as complex as AI, this is easier said than done.... At DeepMind, we start from the premise that all AI applications should remain under meaningful human control and be used for socially beneficial purposes. Understanding what this means in practice requires rigorous scientific inquiry into the most sensitive challenges we face.

So, today we are launching a new research unit, DeepMind Ethics & Society, to complement our work in AI science and application. This new unit will help us explore and understand the real-world impacts of AI. It has a dual aim: to help technologists put ethics into practice and to help society anticipate and direct the impact of AI so that it works for the benefit of all....

During my online exploration on ethics and AI, I found a consensus on the ethical principles that the AI industries have adopted. These are as follows:

1. Aim for the maximum good the AI can do.
2. Identify and eliminate the potential risks in AI design.
3. Use powerful technologies to benefit all societies.

THE CARESSES PROJECT: AN EXAMPLE OF HOW ETHICS CAN BE APPLIED IN ROBOTICS RESEARCH

In terms of how these ethical principles can be used to promote health and eliminate suffering, I am using the *CARESSES* project, which, as I mentioned in other chapters, aimed to develop the first socially assistive and culturally competent robot for the provision of care to older adults primarily residing in care homes. The research team, which included two ethicists, took great care to identify the ethical issues and apply culturally competent solutions. Here are some of the ethical issues listed after a comprehensive literature review (Battistuzzi et al., 2018).

- *Autonomy*: It was ethically important to ensure that interactions with the robot did not reduce participants' sense of autonomy. The research team therefore made it clear to participants during training that they should feel free to reject suggestions for robotic assistance as they wish and that they should contact care staff as they normally would do if they required any care-related support.
- *Culturally determined values and preferences*: The Ethical Guidelines of Alzheimer Europe recognize the importance of respecting and valuing culturally determined priorities and preferences. Thus, the use of the robot should respect and correspond with the cultural traditions of the resident.
- *Dignity and personhood*: Another concern was the possibility that the intervention may serve as an unwanted reminder of diminished personal competencies and independence. Therefore, the software was programmed to ensure that

the direction of interactions and conversations should be determined by the resident rather than the robot. The robot was also programmed to express politeness, praise, and respect of the cultural values of the participants during its interactions, which the researchers hoped would enhance feelings of dignity and self-worth.

- *Privacy*: Sleep and privacy modes were made available, and the participant could also request full privacy, meaning testing and surveillance are paused and the robot removed. Skype calls to the participants were not recorded, conversations generated between the participant and the robot were not stored, and photographs and videos sent via the robot to friends/family were also not stored.
- *Informed consent*: Voluntarily and freely participating in the study with no pressure or coercion was key. Therefore, it was made clear in the information and consent forms, and during recruitment, that there were no penalties for nonparticipation, that participation was completely voluntary, and that the participants could drop out at any time without giving any reason. The informed consent process was culturally sensitive and was not rushed, and residents were encouraged to take time to make their decision over whether to participate or not by talking with their informal caregivers.
- *Preventing harm*: Due to robot's design, the software being used, and the live surveillance, it was viewed as very unlikely that any direct physical harm might take place. The data collection tools used were validated, reliable, and proven to

be acceptable and sensitive. The pretrial pilot also showed no issues. Researchers and technicians were trained to interact sensitively and culturally appropriately.
- *Stigma*: Negative labeling of participants by others (social stigma) or by themselves (self-stigma) was viewed as potentially resulting in harm. Therefore, the study team treated and interacted with participants with dignity, respect, and sensitivity. The researchers and technicians were also trained on these issues to ensure they do not stigmatize (now or in the future). Findings were anonymized and identities protected during dissemination, with the population being addressed with respect and in a nonstigmatizing way.

Protocols for the management of participant distress, incidental findings (i.e., observations or findings that may have occurred during the trial but were unrelated to the specific goals of the trial), and reportable events (i.e., an adverse event or incident that was assessed as being reasonably likely to pose a significant risk to participants or others) were also produced.

Throughout the project and trial, a commitment to maintaining the participants' anonymity and confidentiality during all procedures was made, including during screening, recruitment, testing, evaluation, and dissemination procedures. Data collection, usage, and storage procedures complied with national laws and the EU's General Data Protection Regulation (GDPR) including the commitment for the participants' right to access, right to be informed, right to withdraw, and right to data erasure. Data collection complied with the principle of data minimization, that is, that the collection of personal information from study participants is limited to what is directly relevant and necessary to accomplish the specific goals of the testing and evaluation of work packages. No data related to a third party were stored. This included any audio, video, or sensory data collected upon a person not part of the study, such as a visitor or a staff member, who entered a room during testing. All screening data were deleted upon completion of the project. During the testing procedures, all visual, auditory, and sensory data that the robot collected and processed in order to function as planned were also destroyed after the procedures had been completed. The exception to this was the collection of the number of interactions that the robot logged with each participant. However, these interactions were anonymous. Research data were entered, stored, and managed online through an encrypted and secure Google Drive project account, with only project team members having access to it.

ARISTOTELIAN ETHICS

It is generally acknowledged that modern ethics are rooted in the Aristotelian ethics that emphasize the development of virtues and the pursuit of eudaimonia, which can be translated as flourishing or living a happy life. Simply put, Aristotle's philosophy of ethics was based on the question: *How can we flourish and be happy?* While Aristotle's ethical framework was developed in the context of human behavior, its principles can be applied and adapted to the field of AI ethics and cultural competence in several ways:

Virtue ethics in AI development: Aristotelian virtue ethics suggest that individuals should cultivate virtuous traits such as honesty, integrity, courage, compassion, and a sense of justice. In the context of AI development, this translates into creating systems that embody virtuous characteristics. For example, AI systems should be designed for the common good and prioritize fairness, transparency, accountability, and practical wisdom.

Eudaimonia in AI goals: In the realm of AI ethics, developers and policymakers can apply this concept by ensuring that AI technologies are aligned with human values and contribute positively to the overall well-being of society.

Ethical decision-making in AI: Aristotle's emphasis on practical wisdom (phronesis) can guide the development of AI systems capable of ethical decision-making. Incorporating ethical principles into the algorithms and decision-making processes of AI technologies can contribute to responsible and morally sound outcomes.

Cultural competence and virtue ethics: Aristotle's virtue ethics can be adapted to the development of AI systems with cultural competence. Virtues such as open-mindedness, cultural sensitivity, and inclusivity can be integrated into the design and implementation of AI technologies to ensure they respect and consider diverse cultural perspectives.

Ethical leadership in AI governance: Aristotle's ideas about virtuous leadership can inform the governance of AI technologies. Those responsible for AI development and deployment should embody virtues such as fairness, justice, and responsibility, guiding the ethical use of AI within society.

Context sensitivity: Aristotle recognized the context sensitivity of virtue and that different cultures define ideals differently. This ensures that AI considers different cultural frameworks rather than being narrowly designed around one perspective.

It is important to note that while Aristotelian ethics can provide a philosophical foundation for ethical considerations in AI, the field of AI ethics is multidimensional and involves a combination of ethical theories, legal frameworks, and cultural considerations. Additionally, addressing biases in AI and ensuring cultural competence require a comprehensive approach that considers the diversity of human experiences and values.

Listening to the Voices of Patients and Health Professionals

As healthcare AI and robotics solutions spread, ensuring cultural competence requires ongoing dialogue between innovators, patients, and practitioners locally and globally.

It is essential for developers and researchers in the field of AI robotics in healthcare to engage with patients, healthcare practitioners, and other stakeholders throughout the development process. Involving end users ensures that the technology meets real-world needs, is user-friendly, and addresses ethical and safety concerns. Ongoing participation of these key stakeholders while technologies are researched, piloted, and implemented could prevent failures, such as inaccuracies, irrelevance, safety, and so on. Stakeholders' lived experiences can inform health AI/robotics and result in more successful adoption.

Recently, there has been some criticism of and concerns raised about AI companies accessing large amounts of health data from hospitals and other health-related institutions. For example, Shabani & Marelli (2019) examined the privacy risks around health data and AI with regards to the extensive data access agreements between technology firms and hospital networks. They argued that this level of private health data consolidation into 'data oligopolies' poses risks of exploitation and calls for closer policy scrutiny:

The consolidation of health data in this manner aggravates asymmetries of information and power between data subjects and controllers, thereby increasing exploitation risks.... Policy interventions limiting oligopolistic accumulations of health data may therefore provide the most robust long-term solutions from a welfare perspective.

In another paper from 2021, Vayena and colleagues highlighted public distrust and lack of transparency around some data-sharing partnerships between health systems and AI developers. In their opinion these partnerships highlight the need for responsible data governance, including audits, stronger regulations around transparency and public accountability.

These and other critics (Shabani & Marelli, 2019) highlight concerns about unacceptable practices. It is becoming increasingly more evident that AI robotics companies should actively seek input from diverse patient populations and healthcare workers early and often when researching or designing new AI systems. Setting up participatory committees of patients, families, community leaders, and healthcare workers to provide recommendations and feedback is important, as this will help the technologists progress responsibly and never compromise compassionate care.

Posthuman Perspectives of AI and Culturally Competent Robots

As AI advances, robots and intelligent systems are taking on increasingly sophisticated roles in healthcare, automation, and daily life. Some theorists argue that this proliferation of capable AI constitutes an emerging 'posthuman' era, where technologies expand human capacities and blur boundaries between humans and machines (Ranisch & Sorgner, 2021). However, most AI and robots currently lack cultural competency—the ability to understand and interact appropriately with different human cultures. Providing recommendations misses social nuances or exhibits biases against minority groups (Hagman-Shannon, 2021). Some argue that truly posthuman existence integrates human contexts like culture seamlessly into technological systems. The remainder of this chapter analyzes connections among the rise of culturally competent AI, envisioned posthuman eras, and key associated debates.

DEFINING POSTHUMAN THEORY

Posthuman theory contemplates that advanced technology is radically changing core aspects of human existence. Different streams argue that biological evolution, cognitive enhancement devices, virtual worlds, or AI surpassing human intelligence could trigger a posthuman future (Han, 2021). Common themes include human and machine convergence, technology profoundly expanding capabilities, and redefinitions of life (Graham, 2002). Some proponents like transhumanist philosopher Nick Bostrom argue that deliberate augmentation using biotechnology and machines will direct evolution toward a posthuman condition. Others see posthumanism emerging through technology independently, progressing beyond human control (Lykke, 2021). Overall, the concept remains fluid but centers on technology enabling a step change in physical, mental, and social realities (Ranisch & Sorgner, 2021).

CULTURAL COMPETENCY IN AI AND POSTHUMAN PERSPECTIVES

Cultural gaps significantly impede integration of current AI and robotics systems into human societies. However, some argue that building cultural competency constitutes an early step toward deeper posthuman symbiosis. Tegmark (2017) theorizes AI advancement through four levels: assistive AI enhancing capabilities (L1); AI systems outperforming humans in specialized tasks (L2); theory-of-mind AI rivaling general human competencies (L3); and AI exceeding all human capabilities (L4). Achieving L3 would require AI to relate socially and exhibit cultural competencies comparable to people. Ranisch and Sorgner (2021) similarly argue that cultural awareness indicates higher machine "enculturation" aligning intelligent systems closer with human contexts—a precursor to posthuman existences. Fundamentally integrating culture into AI meaningfully closes human–machine gaps.

Moreover, automated adaptation to individual users' cultural preferences using techniques like deep learning constitutes an embodiment of "transhuman" enhancement—technology personalizing to transcend basic human variation limits (Han, 2021).

KEY DEBATES ON CULTURAL AI AND POSTHUMAN THEORY

Several debates intersect with cultural competency in AI systems and posthuman perspectives.

Can machines achieve cultural capabilities akin to humans? Philosophers like Searle argue that computational processes underpinning AI can never replicate innate human consciousness and understanding essential for relating cross-culturally (Kuflik, 1999). However, modern techniques like consuming training datasets, reinforcement learning, and natural language processing do enable AI to participate broadly in cultural contexts, albeit imperfectly. The line between emulated and authentic cultural awareness remains disputed.

How does cultural bias in AI systems challenge visions of posthuman futures? Existing sociotechnical biases against minority groups in AI development processes undermine narratives of technological convergence with humanity. Resolving biases requires engaging diverse knowledge sources neglected by current developers—achieving this inclusive design is vital for progressing towards posthuman symbiosis (Danks & London, 2017).

Could enhancing cultural competence entrench divisive categories? Critiques argue that explicitly encoding cultural differences for AI utilization risks misrepresenting dynamic identities and ossifying reductive social categories of "culture" reflecting historical power imbalances (Kapuš et al., 2022)—undermining aims for common understanding. However, eschewing culture risks marginalizing minority needs and values. Balancing responsiveness and flexibility remains an open challenge (Jenks, 2011).

Do visceral human reactions against highly capable AI limit human–machine convergence? Theories like the "uncanny valley" argue that when AI closely but imperfectly emulates human characteristics like culture, people instinctively reject it as eerie or untrustworthy. Matching both visible technical competence and nuanced social abilities may be vital for widespread acceptance essential to posthuman integration (Mohammad & Nishida, 2021).

Overall, the path toward culturally competent, enculturated AI holds promise for gradually realizing theorized posthuman futures but remains obstructed by pivotal ethical, social, and technical dilemmas that academic and industry communities continue debating.

Conclusion

The emergence of AI and robotics with increasing abilities to participate appropriately in human cultural contexts aligns with several key premises of posthuman theory—the notion that technology could enable radical advances in mental and social capacities, changing the fundamental nature of existence. Building cultural competency using modern techniques implies a stepping stone toward deeper symbiosis and coevolution between intelligent systems and people-envisioned future states. However, realizing such promise depends on resolving pivotal challenges like biases in AI and potential instinctive rejection of highly enculturated machines. The trajectory of cultural AI competencies will substantially shape progress toward or away from theorized posthuman eras. Issues of transparent and ethical technological design are critical waypoints in this debate. Ultimately, cultural competency marks one axis among many on the complex spectrum between human and machine—but understanding its evolution offers rich insight into society's overall orientation.

Activity

Download one of the free LMs and explore their capabilities and usability by asking the LM three questions about any topic you wish.

Document your reflections on (a) the experience, (b) the accuracy of the information, and (c) potential use.

REFERENCES

Battistuzzi, L., Sgorbissa, A., Papadopoulos, C., Papadopoulos, I., & Koulouglioti, C. (2018). Embedding ethics in the design of culturally competent socially assistive robots. In, *IEEE/RSJ International Conference on Intelligent Robots and Systems (IROS) - Madrid.* Institute of Electrical and Electronics Engineers Inc.

Danks, D., & London, A. J. (2017). Algorithmic Bias in Autonomous Systems. In *IJCAI International Joint Conference on Artificial Intelligence.* https://www.ijcai.org/proceedings/2017/595.

DeepMind blog. https://deepmind.google/discover/blog/why-we-launched-deepmind-ethics-society/

Google: AI Principles Progress Update. https://ai.google/static/documents/ai-principles-2023-progress-update.pdf.

Graham, E. (2002). *Representations of the post/human.* Rutgers University Press.

Hagman-Shannon, B. (2021). Making robots culturally competent. *Science Robotics, 6*(56). https://www.science.org/doi/10.1126/scirobotics.abg3696.

Han, B.-C. (2021). *Entgrenzung: Auf dem Weg in eine posthumanistische Kultur?* Matthes & Seitz Berlin.

Jenks, A. C. (2011). From "lists of traits" to "open-mindedness": Emerging issues in cultural competence education. *Culture, Medicine and Psychiatry, 35*(2), 209–235.

Kapuš, P., Richmond, K., & Jurcík, T. (2022). On posthumanism, bias and ethics of AI systems. *Journal of Artificial Intelligence and Consciousness, 9*(2), 277–302.

Kuflik, A. (1999). Computers in control: Rational transfer of authority or irresponsible abdication of autonomy? *Ethics and Information Technology, 1*(3), 173–184.

Kwoh, Y. S., Hou, J., Jonckheere, E. A., & Hayati, S. (1988). A robot with improved absolute positioning accuracy for CT guided stereotactic brain surgery. *IEEE Transactions on Biomedical Engineering, 35*(2), 153–160. https://doi.org/10.1109/10.1354.

Lanfranco, A. R., Castellanos, A. E., Desai, J. P., & Meyers, W. C. (2004). Robotic surgery: A current perspective. *Annals of surgery, 239*(1), 14–21. https://doi.org/10.1097/01.sla.0000103020.19595.7d.

Lykke, N. (2021). Posthuman knowledge. In R. Braidotti, & S. B. Ortner (Eds.), *Posthuman knowledge* (pp. 319–341). Princeton University Press.

McCarthy J., Minsky M. L., Rochester N., Shannon C.E. (1955). A proposal for the Dartmouth summer research project on artificial intelligence. http://jmc.stanford.edu/articles/dartmouth/dartmouth.pdf

Mohammad, Y., & Nishida, T. (2021). A review on uncanny valley and beyond. *SN Computer Science, 2*(3), 155.

Moyle, W., et al. (2019). Using a therapeutic companion robot for dementia symptoms in long-term care: Reflections from a cluster-RCT. *Aging and Mental Health, 23*(3), 329–336. doi:10.1080/13607863.2017.1421617.

Office of Minority Health. (2013). *National standards for culturally and linguistically appropriate services in health and health care.* U.S. Department of Health and Human Services.

Papadopoulos, I., & Koulouglioti, C. (2022). From stories to scenarios and guidelines for the programming of culturally competent, socially assistive robots. In I. Papadopoulos et al. (Ed.), *Transcultural Artificial Intelligence and robotics in health and social care.* Elsevier Academic Press.

Ranisch, R., & Sorgner, S. L. (2021). *Post- and transhumanism: An introduction.* Routledge.

Shabani, M., & Marelli, L. (2019). Reassessing policy paradigms: A critical reflection on health data governance in the era of big data. *The Information Society, 35*(4), 198–216.

Schwab, K. (2016). The Fourth Industrial Revolution: what it means, how to respond. *World Economic Forum.* https://www.weforum.org/agenda/2016/01/the-fourth-industrial-revolution-what-it-means-and-how-to-respond/.

Tegmark, M. (2017). *Life 3.0: Being human in the age of artificial intelligence.* Knopf.

UNESCO (2018). Preliminary Study on the Ethics of Artificial Intelligence. https://unesdoc.unesco.org/ark:/48223/pf0000265559

UNESCO (2019). Artificial Intelligence and Gender Equality: Key Findings of UNESCO's Global

Dialogue.   https://unesdoc.unesco.org/ark:/48223/pf0000367416

UNESCO (2020). Steering AI and Advanced ICTs for Knowledge Societies: A Rights, Openness, Access, and Multi-stakeholder Perspective. https://unesdoc.unesco.org/ark:/48223/pf0000373434

UNESCO (2021). Recommendation on the Ethics of Artificial Intelligence. https://unesdoc.unesco.org/ark:/48223/pf0000380455

Vayena, E., Blasimme, A., & Cohen, I. G. (2021). What's next for AI in health care. *AMA Journal of Ethics, 23*(2), E105–E110.

Epilogue

As we look to the future, in my opinion, the importance of cultural competence in healthcare will only continue to grow. In a world increasingly marked by conflict, wars, and major health disasters, the ability of healthcare professionals to navigate and respect diverse cultural differences will be more critical than ever.

Technological advancements will undoubtedly shape the future of cultural competence. Telemedicine, artificial intelligence, and virtual reality may offer new ways to bridge cultural gaps and provide culturally sensitive care across distances. However, we must remain vigilant to ensure that these technologies are developed and deployed in an equitable and inclusive manner, avoiding the risk of further marginalizing underserved populations.

Medical discoveries and innovations will also play a significant role. As we gain a deeper understanding of the genetic, epigenetic, and sociocultural factors influencing health, we must integrate this knowledge into culturally competent practices. Personalized and precision medicine hold great promise, but we must ensure that these advancements benefit all populations and do not exacerbate existing health disparities.

Leadership will be key in promoting a culturally competent and virtuous approach to healthcare. We need leaders who recognize the inherent dignity and worth of every individual, regardless of their cultural background; leaders who prioritize compassion, humility, and respect in their interactions with patients, families, and communities; as well as leaders who are willing to challenge systemic inequities and advocate for policies that promote health equity and social justice.

Moreover, we must expand our understanding of cultural competence to encompass the contributions of nonhuman entities. From the microorganisms that inhabit our bodies to the ecosystems that sustain our planet, we are inextricably connected to the natural world. By recognizing the interdependence of human and nonhuman life, we can develop a more holistic and sustainable approach to healthcare.

The future of cultural competence is not without challenges, but it is also full of opportunities. By embracing diversity, equity, and inclusion as core values, by harnessing the power of technology and innovation for the greater good, and by cultivating compassionate and visionary leadership, we can create a more humane and just healthcare system for all. It is a future worth striving for and one that will require the dedication and collaboration of healthcare professionals, researchers, educators, policymakers, and communities around the globe.

Irena Papadopoulos
April 2025

Index

Page numbers followed by *b*, *t*, and *f* indicate boxes, tables, and figures, respectively